EYEBODY

EYEBODY

The Art of Integrating Eye, Brain and Body —
and letting go of glasses forever

Peter Grunwald

EYEBODY PRESS
in association with STEELE ROBERTS

Disclaimer

The names and some details of people mentioned in Chapter 5 have been changed for reasons of personal and professional confidence, but my aim has been to preserve the essence of their story.

The publisher and author of this material make no medical claims for its use. This material is not intended to treat, diagnose, advise about, or cure any illness. If you need medical attention, you are strongly recommended to consult with your registered medical practitioner and you should not rely upon the contents of this publication.

So far as may legally effectively be provided no liability of any kind or nature whatsoever, whether in negligence, under statute, or otherwise, is accepted by the author or the publisher for the accuracy or safety of any of the information or advice contained in, or in any way relating to any part of the content of, this book.

Eyebody® and Eyebody Method® are registered trademarks
Copyright © 2004 Peter Grunwald
Reprinted 2005

National Library of New Zealand Cataloguing-in-Publication Data

Grunwald, Peter, 1958-
Eyebody : the art of integrating eye, brain and body —
and letting go of glasses forever / Peter Grunwald. 2004 ed.
Includes bibliographical references and index.

ISBN 1-877338-41-9

1. Vision. 2. Orthoptics. 3. Mind and body. 4. Brain stimulation.
617.706851—dc 22

Cover design by Micha Wellnitz
Printed by Astra Print, Wellington, New Zealand

First edition, published in 2004 in New Zealand by
Eyebody Press, Box 46 325, Herne Bay, Auckland 1002, New Zealand
in association with Steele Roberts Ltd Publishers, Box 9321 Wellington

Contents

Acknowledgements

Much gratitude and many thanks to all those who have helped in so many ways to support and encourage me in my life, my work, and not least in writing this book.

My appreciation goes to my early teacher, Franz Lohmar. I specially thank Jeremy Chance, Rosemary Chance and William Brenner, the teachers at SATA, Jean Clark, the late Marjory Barstow, my Alexander colleague Penelope Carr, and Zahira Rickard for their support during my Alexander training years.

For my early learning in vision re-education, my gratitude goes to the late Dr Janet Goodrich and Dr Robert-Michael Kaplan.

From my early years in New Zealand discovering the Eye-Body patterns, my thanks go to the late Erna Moss, Guida Lawrence, Louise Gauld, Hanneke Beets and the late Colleen English, to name just a few.

Many thanks to Matthias Erdrich, Galen Cranz, Susanne Stiess, Anja Saunders, Yuzuru Katagiri, Gerlinde Lamprecht, Lucy Ascham, Jeremy Chance, Dagmar Thürnagel, Irene and Christian Sutter-Lukanow, Tara Sullivan, David Moore, Shelley Tibbitts, John Lauer and Sylvie Korkman for their continuing support; and also to Marjory Fern, Linda Franke, Kay Hogan, Brigitte Cavadias, Ron Salazar, Rosa Luisa Rossi and Marianne Moinet.

Rainer Hübner, Hubertus Gerlach, Micha Wellnitz and Martin Kern — your friendship means a huge amount to me. I also want to acknowledge all those friends associated with the Mana Retreat Centre in New Zealand.

With regard to this book, my gratitude goes to Galen Cranz for the foreword, Ellen Webster and Inge Dyson who read the book in its draft form and gave valuable comments, to the professional advice of Dr Jördis Tielsch and behavioral optometrist Mark Grossman, to Alicia Dowsett for her talent in transforming my internal pictures into the drawings accompanying this edition, Micha Wellnitz for the cover design, Martin

Benfell from 20/20 design for the graphics, Hanneke Beets for the colour addition to the Eyebody map, Elaine Russell for typing and Rima Herber for photographs. Many thanks also to Roger Steele and Roger Whelan at Steele Roberts Publishing.

Much gratitude goes especially to Penelope Carroll for her many hours of editorial expertise and support from conception to final completion of this book, and to Tara Sullivan for her time and dedication in refining the underlying principles and contents. Thanks to both of you for your commitment to seeing this book through.

Without understanding and support behind the scenes this book could not have been completed. My deepest love and appreciation goes to my wife Isolde, my children Max and Magdalena for their inquisitive minds and the spark in their eyes, and to my parents Käte and Günter Grunwald, who always believed in and supported me, even in the wildest of times.

And finally to all of you who allowed me to share your experiences and concerns during my retreats, lectures and individual consulting around the world for many years — it is impossible to thank each and every one of you and I hope this book brings encouragement, inspiration, motivation and depth perception.

FOREWORD

In 1999 I attended the International Alexander Congress in Freiburg, Germany to promote my own book, *The Chair: Rethinking Culture, Body and Design*. There I was told that the most interesting presenter was Peter Grunwald, so I joined a standing-room-only crowd to hear him. He was talking about eyes (switching freely between English and German, sometimes in the same sentence!) but my vision was fairly good. He asked a volunteer with a vision problem to 'lengthen and widen her cornea.' Later a medically trained friend assured me that doing anything to a structure without voluntary muscles was impossible. Nevertheless, like most of the other Alexander teachers in the audience, I readily followed his directions. To my surprise, a couple of vertebrae in my back shifted more to the midline.

As the crowd thinned I waited to speak to Peter, explaining that I had followed his directions but that my spine moved. "Oh," he said, "that's because that part of the eye governs that part of the body." Obviously he had worked something out about the eye and the body. Oh no, I thought; yet another system I will have to investigate. He was far too busy with others for me to press him for more information, but internally I noted that I would work with him if I ever got the opportunity. When it comes to finding ways to unlock the mystery of scoliosis, I leave no stone unturned.

One of the 'stones' I turned over two decades earlier was the Alexander Technique, a system of posture and movement developed by an Australian at the end of the 19th century. It has allowed me to flourish despite what the medical world would consider a crippling curvature of 80 degrees. In fact, it has allowed me to reduce this curvature despite the medical expectation that it would worsen one degree per year. The technique works because it involves the whole self, the mind as well as the body.

Early in 2000 I heard that Peter would offer his first American workshop in California, so I signed up. On the basis of that first six-day experience I learned that in searching for ways to transform his own myopia, astigmatism, and stuttering, Peter had synthesized the Alexander Technique and the Bates Method of Natural Vision, primarily to teach people how to see without using glasses or contacts. I realized that he had done significantly more than synthesize the two techniques; he has transcended both, creating a new method of body-mind integration.

This first workshop with Peter was a series of 'aha' experiences, culminating in the certainty that in his use of vision I had found a missing link. At last, a concrete, step-by-step way to move from the mental to the physical, from the physical to the mental — through imagination and the brain itself! Peter was offering a way to go into a serene state and directly perceive in 3-D without elaborate brainwave feedback equipment — through my own visual pathway. The potential was clear to me and I knew that this was the next step in my psycho-physical-spiritual development for the next several years.

I had come to Peter's work knowing a fair amount about how the mind interacts with the body because of nearly 30 years of exploration as a scholar, client, and practitioner in what have come to be known as 'somatic practices,' defined as the relationship between body, thought, cultural belief, individual feeling and will. BodyMind Centering (BMC) emphasizes the importance of 'experiential anatomy,' the idea — no, the experience! — of being able to enter an anatomical structure mentally. Behavioural optometry maintains that eyesight can change, and I experienced this myself; through vision training, I overcame a small convergence deficiency, regained the flexibility of my lens so that I did not have to start wearing bifocals at 45, and eventually regained my 20/20 vision.

How might vision training relate to such somatic themes? Peter starts with vision as the path into body, culture, feeling and will. He argues that our culture has become excessively focused on detail and clarity and that we have lost the practice of keeping peripheral vision open to see the big picture. When we were hunters and gatherers, staying connected to the big picture of form and movement was just as important as getting the details right.

Three-dimensional images are produced in the brain, not out in the eyes. Our brains do this for us automatically, but if we choose to think about the process consciously, as Peter teaches us, then vision pops into three dimensions in an especially vivid way. Instead, most of the time we *interpret* two-dimensional vision as having perspective. The direct perception of three-dimensionality is startling, fresh, and, in the old-fashioned sense, awesome. As a poet has said, *Seeing is forgetting the name of the thing one sees.* This is one goal of meditative practice — to move toward pure perception. Peter's method offers a practical spirituality.

I have continued to work with Peter ever since that first workshop, including travelling to New Zealand every January to participate in the 3-week workshops he organizes for intensive study. Occasionally a friend might ask why I take the same workshop over and over; haven't I learned it by now? I would liken it to music camp, where you go to practise even though you might already know the songs you intend to play. With practise we get better — more confident and more competent. A worldwide network is developing, linking friends in New Zealand, Australia, the United Kingdom, Germany, Switzerland, Austria, Sweden, France, the United States, South Africa and Japan. Members of this emerging community support one another in pursuit of this path toward wholeness. Peter has a gift, which he is willing to share. Therefore he remains central to this community, and I am happy to say that he supports its ongoing evolution into a network, rather than a centralized organization. I expect that ageing in the company of this group should be interesting and supportive. One of the highest and best uses of his method that I can foresee for myself — besides the creation of a magnificently upright, wide, and full torso — is to be able to die consciously and beautifully. Here I imagine these friends will help each other by consciously staying 'in depth.'

By now you may have rightly inferred that the Eyebody Method has applications for those who have other issues not directly related to eyesight. The most practical tool is the idea that the visual pathway — all the way from the front of the eye up to the visual cortex — is a model of the human body and that different parts of the eye correspond to different parts of the body. Perhaps even more powerful is the idea that once we learn how to see in depth consciously we can shape our future. This is what some philosophers have termed 'emergence,' where the future shapes the past, the envisioned shapes our present.

The mechanism by which these things happen remain beyond current scientific understanding, but they may become better understood in the future since the scientific community is paying more attention to the relationships between subjectivity and objectivity. No matter what science ends up confirming, what is for certain and important is that Peter has offered a practical technique for working with the powers of your mind.

Those who meditate may recognize his directions as a way to get to the experience of serenity, clarity, acceptance, beauty, and perfection. It can be used by all kinds of people. Glasses are not necessarily the issue, but rather regaining and securing the ability to see, think and feel in three dimensions.

This work has important implications for architects and designers. Instead of *interpreting* two-dimensional vision as having perspective, designers especially would benefit from *perceiving* three-dimensionally. Consciously choosing depth perception affects physical sight, emotion, and judgment — all essential to creativity in architectural design. My colleagues in environmental design research will appreciate that once when I was consciously using my visual cortex I was able to experience directly the personal space bubbles that the anthropologist Edward Hall described as surrounding each individual. I believe that if architects and planners could more directly experience three-dimensionality, they might be able to champion radiant human settlements, in contrast to the dreary, soulless contemporary built environments, shaped so much by 'the bottom line.' In regard to my own specialty I would hope that furniture and interior designers would be able to appreciate seating design as a three-dimensional problem, not a two-dimensional graphic problem regarding which chair looks best in a setting. Envisioning the pleasure and beauty of body-conscious design will help them reject the stresses imposed by a roomful of chairs and tables that perpetuate the classic right-angle seated posture.

Peter's method works at several levels: physical, emotional, intellectual, and spiritual. Although I came to this work for scoliosis, I have stayed because of the pleasure found in my own brain. That is not to say that my scoliosis has not changed; on my last trip back from New Zealand in January 2004 my osteopath commented on how much less twisted my upper spine is. Others are exploring various eye conditions, new ways to think about and teach the Alexander Technique, and general habits of mind. The applications are numerous and continuously evolving. This book is not a history of a finished work, but rather a first report on an evolving art. It is an invitation to participate.

Galen Cranz, Ph D, STAT, AmSAT
Professor of Social Architecture, University of California at Berkeley
31 May 2004
Oakland, CA

Discovering eye, brain and body connections

Wearing glasses was for me a way of life — and a burden! I grabbed them as soon as I got out of bed, I used them while showering (was I checking to see whether I was really wet?), I needed them for getting dressed, and at school for both close-up reading and to see the blackboard clearly. I used special frames for swimming, running and other sports and they got in the way when I was first dating. I was totally dependent on them. I never questioned whether I could function without glasses; it never entered my mind.

I seemed to be equally dependent on stuttering and poor breathing, on my slumped posture and sore back. I was filled with a constant sense of anxiety. Certainly all my efforts to correct my stuttering came to nothing — in fact it got progressively worse. It never occurred to me that there might be links between my short-sightedness and astigmatism and my speech and breathing problems, my poor posture and back problems, the all-pervasive sense of anxiety I felt — and even my inability to learn and retain information.

To avoid compulsory military service in Germany I trained my eyes to get worse — and went through two pairs of increasingly strong lenses within six months, in the end getting what I wanted: I was exempted from military service because of my eyesight.

If I was able to worsen my eyes, was it possible to learn how to improve them? Years later I started to explore this and found the answer was 'yes'. I am very grateful for the guidance of the late Dr Janet Goodrich (1942–1999), whose teaching combined the Bates Method, principles of Reichian therapy and Brain Gym activities. Through my work with her I was able to free myself of prescription lenses in just 18 months — and from there discovered the links between my short-sightedness and lower back pain, my astigmatism and speech disability.

Being able to let go of glasses — although enormously freeing in itself

— was only the beginning. One day in 1992 I became physically aware of my cornea and acutely aware of sensation there. I found I could tighten and relax my cornea at will and noticed that my chest area responded. When I tightened my cornea my chest tightened and slumped. When I thought of releasing my cornea, my upper body started to straighten up and lengthen out and my breathing improved markedly. As long as I was 'in' my cornea I could do this over and over again, without fail. It was years before I understood the full significance of this experience.

In the years that followed I discovered that within the visual system resides a map of the human body in its entirety. I call this the *Eyebody Patterns*. The eyes themselves are similarly linked to corresponding structures in the brain. In addition, the visual system, including the eyes and their supporting neural structures, contains links to our autonomic nervous system (the reptilian brain), our emotions (the limbic brain) and our ability to think and reason (the neocortex).

Seeing is much more than meets the eyes. In fact, we do not see with our eyes; seeing happens in the brain. The eyes are merely the organs the brain uses to receive light.

All visual dysfunctions, like short-sightedness, far-sightedness, astigmatism, middle-aged vision (where your arms become too short to read the newspaper), glaucoma, cataracts and crossed-eyes can be traced back to corresponding dysfunctions in the eyes, body, and brain.

Many years experience with thousands of people in workshops, small groups and private sessions has confirmed the reliability of the interconnecting patterns, and enabled me to help people like you coordinate and integrate their entire visual system.

By consciously connecting the various components of the visual system, eye, brain and body functions become integrated. This strengthened visual system not only changes the physical structures of the eye over time but also integrates emotional, mental and spiritual aspects of our being. As the visual system becomes more coordinated the need for glasses or contact lenses is lessened and eventually disappears — glasses can become a thing of the past.

Let us find some common ground before I take you on this journey of discovery. We begin from the standpoint that as human beings we can operate at our highest potential by not interfering with our own natural functioning — optimal functioning is part of our natural mechanism.

By natural I mean 'in accordance with nature', or 'as nature intended', not habitual. Most of us get into habits that may or may not benefit us.

Our habits seem 'natural' to us, but that may not be the case. For change in counterproductive habits to occur there has to be an awareness and understanding of what we are doing — and where we would like to go. In terms of vision, this means understanding how we can function in a more efficient, effective, holistic way.

Our brains have the capacity to think outside our habitual patterns. What we usually call 'thinking' occurs in the frontal lobes of the neocortex and is what I call 'two-dimensional thinking'. But there is another sort of 'thinking' that has its origins toward the back of the neocortex, an area I call the upper visual cortex. I associate this area with conscious, three-dimensional thinking. By activating this kind of thinking from this part of the brain I am able to apply my mind in a non-habitual way. Changing habits is, as you probably well know, not easy. It requires commitment. But we can learn to use our brain in a different way.

To illustrate what I mean by commitment, imagine you are in a new partnership. At first there is the honeymoon phase, and any frustrations or criticisms of your partner are overlooked. Then little things can start to bother you. Commitment is needed to overcome these ups and downs. As one workshop participant in France succinctly put it: "Commitment is doing what I said I would do, long after the feeling I had when I said it has passed." Feelings change constantly; commitment can continue to grow as the process unfolds.

The ideas of Frederick Mathias Alexander (1869–1955), whose work has made a vital contribution to humanity, have been integral in the development of my own method and personal process. Part of my earlier professional training was to become a teacher of the Alexander Technique. Alexander, an actor, solved a voice problem through observation and mental direction. He went on to apply the same techniques to improve other difficulties like poor posture and concentration. Through my work with the Alexander Technique I started observing my own habits of thinking and doing in relationship to the process of seeing.

I also wish to acknowledge the work of William H Bates (1860–1931), a New York ophthalmologist whose work is the precursor of modern natural vision improvement methods. His willingness to question the need for glasses and even visual dysfunction itself opened up a debate which continues to this day.

In a sense I am continuing on a journey begun by writer Aldous Huxley (1894–1963). A seeker of truth in many modalities, Huxley was a student of both Alexander and the Bates method. In his elegant, comprehensive book *The Art of Seeing*, he synthesizes Alexander's principles and Bates' practical methodology and belief system in a way which seems so natural that it comes as a shock that such thinking continues to be unorthodox over half a century later.

My findings come out of years of personal experiences and investigations in experiential anatomy and physiology. I am not a neurologist or neuroscientist, nor am I medically trained. I hope that in years to come scientific studies will be undertaken to support the validity of my findings. But meanwhile let's explore what I have learned working with myself and with the thousands of people I have seen from many different backgrounds, cultures and countries.

This book was inspired by many of my students and clients, who wanted to read more about my developing work and by numerous people interested in the subject even though they had never experienced first hand the processes involved.

The first edition of this book provides an overview both for the interested reader and those already engaged with the Eyebody Method. It may also offer some insights to my colleagues working in the field of eyesight and vision improvement and somatics. It is a work in progress. As I continue to discover new relationships and deepen my understanding, my findings will be included in subsequent editions.

1

A personal story: Letting go of glasses forever

Let me tell you how I threw away my glasses, learned to see naturally and came to understand the connections between eye, brain and body.

I was born in Germany in the late 1950s. When I was three my mother — noticing I frequently tripped over — took me to an eye specialist. Poor eyesight runs in the family; both my mother and father are short-sighted and astigmatic. So, it turned out, was I. There I was, at age three, with my first glasses — those little ones for little children. Aside from being stuck behind a pair of specs, I was stuttering badly too. Apparently I took a long time to learn to talk, and when I did, it all came out in a jumble.

The glasses became progressively stronger and thicker. Sometimes I needed two new prescriptions a year. How I dreaded those visits: being seated in front of a monstrous machine, the cold drops which made everything blurry… I felt so vulnerable, and somehow invaded. "Is this line clearer?" the specialist would ask as he changed the lenses. I'd quickly say: "Yes, that's clearer" — anything to be finished and out of there!

Now imagine me as a teenager, stuttering, and boxed in by glasses. My posture had started to slump, with the lower back curved and the shoulders narrowed in. I had learned to manage in life without being able to see or speak clearly — things most of us take for granted. Do you know anybody who stutters? The problem with stuttering is that the listener knows what you want to say before you get it out. It wasn't easy for me to relate to friends. I restricted my friendships to people who had enough patience to wait for me to speak. Others I avoided.

If I can make my eyesight worse, can I improve it too?

In those days military service in Germany was compulsory for males. I was nearing 18, the usual age for going into the army, but being a pacifist, didn't want to enlist. My older brother told me that if his vision had been a bit worse he could have avoided military service. Maybe I could get out of it that way, I thought… but a visit to the eye specialist assured me my vision was adequate. As my birthday came closer I became quite depressed and collapsed in my body. I wrote the appropriate letters to appeal for a social service exemption and at the same time began consciously trying to make my vision worse. In six short months I succeeded; I had to have two new prescriptions as my vision went from bad to worse.

Finally the dreaded day came for the army medical examination. I was nervous and shy as I waited with a bunch of other guys my age. The eye test came first. Immediately afterwards the optometrist said, "I'm really sorry, but you cannot be accepted with such poor eyesight." It was like winning the lottery! The months of slumping and feeling sorry for myself disappeared instantly. I was given an official letter stating I was unable, on account of my vision, to perform military service. When I inquired about alternative social service duties I was told that if I didn't qualify for the army I would not qualify for social service either. On the way home I suddenly thought, if I can train my vision to get worse, perhaps I can improve it, too? But you know how youngsters are. It was years before I gave any further thought to improving my eyesight.

I completed my formal education and set off travelling: Europe, the Middle East, North Africa and then India. If you have visited India you know how different from the Western way of life everything there is. The Indian sense of the spiritual, especially the daily submersion in prayers and worship, was extraordinary to a young German traveller. After several months there I became very sick — nothing unusual in India. My stomach didn't know whether it was up or down, and my intestines and liver didn't like the experience either. It took months to recuperate from hepatitis, resting up in a little hut on the beach. I drank nothing but boiled water and ate only a little rice and fresh fruit. My nervous system slowed down tremendously. It was as if I was letting go of the accumulation of years of frenetic Western life. I ended up feeling refreshed and energized, and well enough to travel again.

The extraordinary art of seeing

As I settled into the last seat on a local bus, something very strange happened. Seeing from the back of my skull and the middle of my brain, my surroundings became completely clear and three-dimensional and the colours extraordinarily vivid; I felt I was seeing inside people and clearly perceiving their true nature. I experienced a wonderful mental clarity. I was completely connected, merging with this 3-D world. It was an experience I was not able to switch off even if I had wanted to. I felt peaceful and calm, yet emotionally totally present and alive. This experience lasted the rest of the day.

Next morning this way of seeing and being was still as fresh and alive as the previous day. Whatever it was, it persisted for months and I enjoyed every moment of it. Every day I woke with this clarity of vision, thought and focus, and a heightened awareness of myself and my environment. No sense of fear, anxiety or anguish, no wandering thoughts, no judgements of myself or others. During this time I felt fearless, yet extraordinarily loving, kind and well connected. I felt totally present, content with myself and my surroundings. It was a completely mind-altering experience — without drugs. I was in slow motion, seeing both the big picture and the little details at the same time. I was still stuttering, I was still slumping, and I was still completely reliant on my glasses, but somehow my awareness transcended these shortcomings. One morning I woke up knowing I would one day see clearly without my glasses. It was a very deep sense of knowing: *One day I will be able to see.*

I continued my travels in Asia, still seeing with this heightened sense of awareness, fearless and at peace. Then one day it ended as abruptly as it had begun. I was resting on a hilltop and had closed my eyes to focus on the sounds around me. When I opened my eyes minutes later, everything had changed. The sense of aliveness and connectedness I had felt only moments before had gone. Gone with the flick of an eyelid. How could this happen? And why? I was flooded with emotions. I felt angry and betrayed. All my old fears and anxieties had returned. I cried.

Months of grief followed. I came to really understand the saying, 'the higher you go the farther you fall.' At the time I had no idea the impact the experiences of the previous seven months would have on my entire life: that I would one day learn to consciously access this quality of seeing and that I would teach the techniques to others.

By the time I reached New Zealand I'd been on the road for three years. I was tired of travelling and decided to stay.

Out of the slump and into the Alexander teacher training

The couple caught my eye at a healing festival. They had something in their walk — grace, lightness and lift that I certainly didn't have. I told them, stuttering, how much I admired their walking style. To my surprise they immediately commented on my stuttering. People were usually too polite to comment, and I had managed to avoid thinking about my stuttering for years. They told me that if I read a book called *The Use of the Self* by FM Alexander I would find clues to manage my stuttering, as well as improve my walking and general coordination. I went to the library and borrowed the book. I didn't understand a lot of it, partly because my English was still in its infancy. But I was intrigued by the chapter on stuttering, where Alexander wrote about helping someone to overcome stuttering and improve his general health. I wanted to know more.

A few months later I was in Sydney, Australia, attending a weekend workshop on the Alexander Technique. I was fascinated. By the end of the weekend I felt much freer sitting, standing and walking, and my back ached far less. I also felt a tingle of anticipation: maybe there was something in the Alexander principles which could take me back to that longed-for way of seeing and state of being I had experienced in India. In India it had just happened, but maybe I could find my way there again, step-by-step…

A few weeks later I had started the three year Alexander Technique teacher training. A journalist who interviewed me for an article about the technique a couple of months into our training asked why I was participating. I told her I hoped the technique would help me overcome my lifelong stutter. A few days later her article was published in the *Sydney Morning Herald*. She mentioned me in the article, concluding that the work had already helped me, as I had hardly stuttered during the interview. When I read this I realized how much my speech had improved without my noticing, and I felt much more at ease communicating with people. The impulse to stutter was still there, but it had lessened and over time the pattern dissolved more and more.

How did this happen? Remember I was slumping really badly: this meant my voice box was being pressed down and my whole structure and gut area was slumped and tight. The Alexander Technique helped me recognize this and undo the downward slumping. This in turn allowed my whole body, including my voice, to function as it should.

During my training, the American Alexander teacher Marjory Barstow (1899–1997), who visited Australia for a month every year, became a source of inspiration. She was then in her late 80s and still very dynamic. She had an extraordinary ability to communicate Alexander principles with clarity and understanding and some of her communication skills are very much present with me to this day.

After graduating from the three year Sydney training I stayed on to work with William Brenner and Rosemary Chance. I learned a great deal about working in groups and presenting to large audiences. This time was vital in the development of my speech.

The conscious experience of the blur

One day in 1989 I decided I wanted a pair of contact lenses. With contacts no one would know I couldn't see properly, so I went and got a prescription. But in the days of waiting for them I began to ask myself whether it might be possible to improve my eyesight the way I had my speech and posture. My experience in India came flooding back to me — the sureness of that moment when I knew one day I would see clearly without my glasses. I felt once again the truth of it.

The following weekend I attended a fundamental course in Natural Vision Improvement lead by Dr Janet Goodrich. I was filled with doubts. Was it really possible to improve severe myopia and astigmatism? I had only 40 percent vision in my right eye with the strongest lenses and my left eye was only marginally better. Could I reduce the strength of my glasses — perhaps do without them altogether? The room was full, everyone with different vision problems. Some had been myopic from early childhood, others needed reading glasses for presbyopia after turning 40; some were coping with squints or the effects of eye operations in their youth, others were considering eye surgery; there were participants with astigmatism, glaucoma, cataracts and retinitis pigmentosa. Here were a whole range of visual malfunctions gathered in one big room.

In the first few minutes Janet asked us to take our glasses off. "Welcome to the blur," she said. And she was right. I could only see 10 centimetres in front of my face. The rest was a total blur. I could distinguish no colours or forms, only light and darkness. I felt alone in the room, totally cut off from everything and everybody, yet with a strong sense that here was something to learn, something connected to that previous knowledge that one day I would see without my glasses. The weekend was one of many discoveries, not the least being an experience of my own eyes. I had had no sense of the eyes behind my glasses! That first weekend workshop was certainly an 'eye opener' to me…

The first day without glasses

On the Monday after the workshop I was sitting calmly in the suburban train taking me to the Alexander studio at Milson's Point across Sydney Harbour Bridge, when I suddenly went into shock. I felt paralysed and bewildered. I realized I had forgotten my glasses! For the first time in my life I had forgotten my glasses. I must have gotten out of bed without putting glasses on my nose. I must have had my shower without my glasses, I must have breakfasted without them, walked to the train station and caught the right train in the right direction without them — and found an empty seat on the train in rush hour. All of this without even thinking about glasses or being in the blur. Well, I was certainly aware of the blur now! I would have to go back and get them. Then I calmed down and remembered my intention to see naturally without glasses: I would continue on my day's journey without them. I spent the 40-minute train trip busily 'palming' and 'sunning', two of the vision activities I had just learned. But acute anxiety and fear kept surfacing. I felt naked and vulnerable without my glasses.

If you have ever taken a train over Sydney Harbour Bridge you will know that the train clatters as it crosses the bridge. That was my sign to hop out at the next station. I hurtled down the carriage, waiting in my blurriness for the door to open. Then I had to negotiate the steps on to the platform. I don't think I have ever walked down steps so consciously. Every step was a new experience. Leaving the station, I hugged the shop walls until I reached a flower shop, stopping there to get my bearings. I knew I had to conquer the next 30 metres to reach the pedestrian crossing; the studio was on the other side of a busy road. When I finally arrived at the crossing all I could see were dark moving shadows. I was acutely aware of danger and decided to wait and cross with someone else. I noticed someone standing beside me, then suddenly they were gone. I directed all my attention on the next person who came up beside me. This time I was ready and made it safely across the road. The usual five-minute walk to my studio had taken 20 — but I had made it.

Later in the day a colleague mentioned she had seen me at the pedestrian crossing and that I had seemed strange. What was I doing? I explained what had happened and my commitment to see without glasses. Only a few of my students commented on the absence of my glasses. Some people noticed how pale I was around the rims of my eyes.

During phone conversations that day I realised I was unable to hear clearly. I wondered how seeing and hearing could be associated.

By the end of the day I was totally exhausted, but very pleased too. The whole day had been filled with new experiences and different perspectives. My commitment not to wear glasses grew. It was pleasurable to rediscover mundane activities in a fresh way. It meant staying awake and being creative.

The process of letting go: transition glasses

It was 18 months before I no longer needed my glasses. I had gone back to the optometrist for 'transition glasses', as Dr Goodrich called them, rather than proceed with contact lenses. Transition glasses are reduced in dioptres, safe and legal to drive with, and support the vision improvement process by giving the retina and fovea centralis more freedom to function. The problem with contact lenses is that once they are in, that's it — they stay in all day, or even for a few days. Glasses have the advantage of at least being readily removable. I needed to 'sell' the idea of the transition glasses to the optometrist. When I left with a pair about 2.25 dioptres weaker than the ones I had gone in with, he said, "you are the first person I've had in my shop who hasn't wanted to see clearly!"

The glasses were indeed blurry to look through in the beginning. But by the end of the first week I was amazed at how clearly I could see with them. In just one week my eyes and vision had dramatically improved.

The next step was buying a chain from the pharmacy to hang my glasses around my neck. Removing them frequently allowed my eyes to rest, avoiding the constant staring through the centre point of the lenses and giving my natural vision a chance to be active. Gradually I came to a point where it was pleasant to be without glasses. When I wanted to see particularly clearly I treated myself and put them on. I had to remember to keep taking them off rather leave them on out of habit. This process helped me to become aware of when I needed to wear glasses, when I didn't need them, and when I wished to wear them. It made me aware that I had a choice.

During the process of letting go of my prescription glasses I used pinhole glasses regularly as a tool for intrinsic eye exercise. Pinhole glasses have little holes stamped into black plastic 'lenses'. They allowed me to see clearly watching TV or movies, reading or writing, while at the same time exercising the inside of my eyes.

Walking down the road without glasses was interesting. If I thought I saw someone I knew I would try and work out who it was, then put on my glasses to confirm. After some weeks my guess rate was high, yet I still felt I had to put on those specs to make sure I was right. I realised how closely related trust and vision are. It was time to change the habit of doubting what I saw and leave my glasses off.

As the process of letting go of glasses continued both my physical and mental vision improved, assisted by two months of intensive professional training in Vision Improvement with Dr Goodrich in Germany. During this training I visited an optometrist for a lens reduction. The optometrist couldn't believe what she saw; the reading on her machine was different from what I could actually see on the reading chart, she said repeatedly. This couldn't be the case... By the time she came round to accepting the difference it was lunchtime. Traditionally every shop in rural Germany breaks for lunch from noon to 2.30 p.m., and I arranged to return after lunch to finish the tests. When I returned I felt sleepy and was a little slumped. The optometrist was annoyed that I could not read what I had been able to read in the morning.

In the end I left without a new prescription. I experienced how eyesight fluctuates and changes in response to many stimuli. I have learned to detect these fluctuations, notice changes and apply principles to improve where I am at any given moment. This is a step-by-step approach, bringing step-by-step success.

After my professional vision training I returned to New Zealand. Friends of mine had been building a remarkable centre for adult learning, the Mana Retreat Centre on the Coromandel Peninsula, and we regularly played volleyball there. At that time I was a liability because I could see only a metre without my glasses, which I didn't wear. Some of my friends would say, "Why don't you put glasses on?" or make other comments which certainly didn't support my vision-improving process. I had to avoid the trap of doing what other people thought I should do. Creating healthy boundaries was crucial, otherwise these passing comments could cause me to abandon my original intentions and lead to a feeling of 'I'm not good enough' or 'I can't do this'.

How easy it is to abandon a good intention and continue with an old habit. How easy for paralysing fear or anxiety to creep in. During my vision improvement process I had a sense of changing fear into fearlessness by remaining motivated and committed. And, day by day, step-by-step I succeeded. My vision and volleyball playing improved rapidly and consistently and the comments ceased. I felt inspired.

The commitment to let go of glasses completely

A few months later I made the next big leap. I took the transition glasses off the chain around my neck, put them in a case and stored it in my pocket. Now the glasses weren't so readily available. It took at least five seconds to fiddle around and get them out of the case and onto my nose. Five seconds for a short-sighted person who likes things done instantly is a long time — about the same time it took to focus on and see an object without my glasses. The lesson was to stop and see, rather than have my glasses do the seeing for me. The process became easier and easier.

The day came when I was ready for the supermarket test. I wanted to buy groceries without using my glasses. This was quite a test because, as you know, supermarkets have row upon row of thousands of products, most of which you will never buy. I drove to the supermarket and left the glasses in their case in the car. I knew I had to be creative to get what I wanted. In my mind I started to visualize the butter, bread and milk. I used my vision actively, found the items easily, placed them in my trolley, walked to the cashier, paid for the items and left. From then on I was confident to go shopping without glasses.

As the process continued I recommitted to my intention daily, and sometimes several times a day. I didn't need glasses for any of the activities I enjoyed. And what are 18 months in relation to 27 years of being completely dependent on glasses every day?

In 1991 I let go of my glasses forever. At first my eyesight and vision fluctuated but they stabilized when I discovered and worked with the connections integrating eye, brain and body functions. For over a decade this journey of discovery has continued.

2

How vision works — the Eyebody Patterns

Let me take you on a little journey inside your head, in fact inside your eyes and parts of your brain. It's good to get an overview of how it looks in there, so you can understand and appreciate the system we are addressing — a system which you and I are constantly using. It will help you understand terminology I use throughout the book and give you an overall understanding of how eyesight works according to the conventional medical model.

It's the brain that sees, not the eyes!

The eyes do not see; it is the brain that sees. The eyes are organs that gather visual information for the brain, much in the same way that our hands gather tactile information which the brain then interprets.

There are six characteristics of vision: depth perception, colour, movement, light and darkness, and shape, all of which are processed in the visual part of the brain, which is called the visual cortex.

The three brains

During the evolutionary process we developed three distinct brains (see figure 2.1). First we developed the reptilian brain, the one we share with all vertebrates. I use the term 'reptilian brain' throughout the book to mean the brainstem, third ventricle and the diencephalon, on which we find the thalamus and hypothalamus with their related pineal and pituitary glands, as well as the lateral geniculate bodies — all structures relevant to the visual system (see figure 2.2). It is in the reptilian brain that we find the coordinating processes that make our body function.

Further on in evolution, the limbic system developed. The limbic brain wraps around the reptilian brain. I define the limbic brain throughout this book as the structures immediately surrounding the diencephalon (the 'mushroom hood' of the brainstem) and relevant to the visual system:

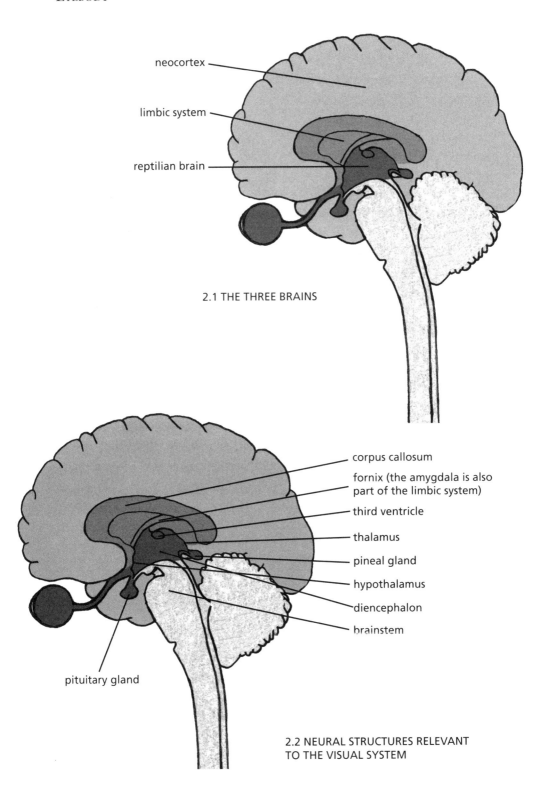

2.1 THE THREE BRAINS

neocortex

limbic system

reptilian brain

corpus callosum

fornix (the amygdala is also
part of the limbic system)

third ventricle

thalamus

pineal gland

hypothalamus

diencephalon

brainstem

pituitary gland

2.2 NEURAL STRUCTURES RELEVANT
TO THE VISUAL SYSTEM

the amygdala, fornix, the limbic fluid, and the lower two-thirds of the corpus callosum. It is also called 'the emotional brain' as it houses our emotional memories.

The neocortex is our most recently developed brain. It is our 'conscious' brain and has helped us get to the moon, build submarines and develop strategic business plans. It is the brain that lets us choose what to do and when to do it. The visual brain is part of the neocortex.

Over time our brain evolved by building on what came before. Each 'brain' has a certain primary function — physical, emotional and mental respectively. The visual system passes through each one of those brains, and is perhaps the only sense that is present in all of them. This is part of what makes the visual system unique, and perhaps why we are primarily visual beings.

As an indication of how remarkably intricate this entire system is, scientists have so far been unable to transplant the retina of a donor to another person's eye. Yet hearts, kidneys, livers and lungs, and even the cornea (on the outer part of the eye) can be transplanted. Connecting the retina to the wiring of the brain has not yet been achieved because of the myriad neural pathways involved.

The visual brain

The visual cortex is at the back of the skull and takes up about a quarter to a third of the entire neocortex (see figure 2.3). A lot of our brain capacity is used for visual processing. You can measure the visual cortex with the palm of your hand; it's approximately 10 centimetres high, 6 centimetres wide and 4 to 5 centimetres deep (see figure 2.4).

2.3 THE VISUAL CORTEX

The visual cortex is constantly sending messages to other areas of the brain, with about 60% of the entire brain involved in visual processing. Brain pathways are activated by every visual thought we have. The visual cortex is responsible not only for eyesight, but also for other aspects of vision: visual memory, visual imag-

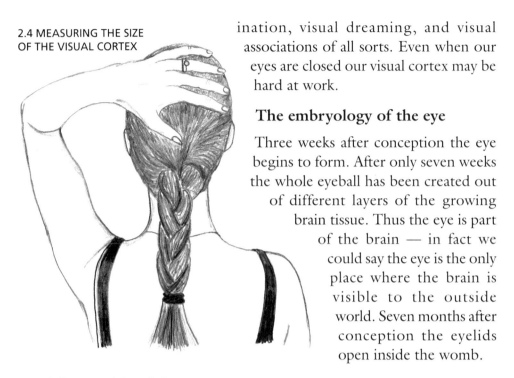

2.4 MEASURING THE SIZE OF THE VISUAL CORTEX

ination, visual dreaming, and visual associations of all sorts. Even when our eyes are closed our visual cortex may be hard at work.

The embryology of the eye

Three weeks after conception the eye begins to form. After only seven weeks the whole eyeball has been created out of different layers of the growing brain tissue. Thus the eye is part of the brain — in fact we could say the eye is the only place where the brain is visible to the outside world. Seven months after conception the eyelids open inside the womb.

The outside of the eye

The external layer of the eye consists of tough sclera. Extrinsic eye muscles, connected to the sclera, move the eye from side to side, up and down — movements we can see easily externally. The eye sits in a fatty fluid for protection and ease of movement (see figure 2.5).

The auxiliary area of the eyes (see figure 2.6) consists of the conjunctiva that is layered between the cornea and the eyelid. The eyelashes connect to the eyelids. The upper tear ducts (lachrymal glands) allow tear fluid to be produced and the lower nasal tear ducts allow the fluid to be secreted.

The anatomy and physiology of the eye

Sight works by means of light passing through the delicate layers of the cornea (see figure 2.7). The light goes through the aqueous humour (the fluid in the frontal area of the eye), through the pupil, the lens and all the way through the vitreous humour (the fluid inside the eye) onto the retina. The retina consists of at least ten layers of photoreceptors called rods and cones. There seems to be no clear consensus as to the specific roles of the rods and cones. One thing that is agreed upon is that the cone photoreceptors are somehow responsible for high-resolution,

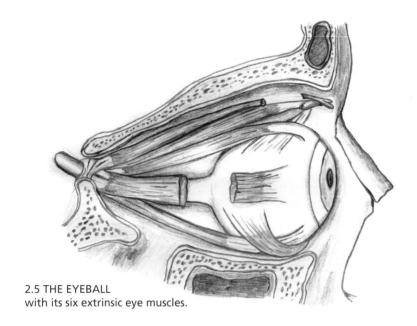

2.5 THE EYEBALL
with its six extrinsic eye muscles.

focused sight and colour perception. Cones are found within the fovea centralis and the macula which surrounds it; this area is responsible for detailed vision. The rod photoreceptors are situated in the peripheral area of the retina beyond the edge of the macula, all the way up to the ora serrata, the 'serrated edge' where the photoreceptors end (towards the front of the eye). It is generally believed that rods are responsible for night vision and peripheral seeing. The layer of the retina extends past the ora serrata all the way to the inside of the pupil; the retinal layer continues, but this frontal part contains no photoreceptors.

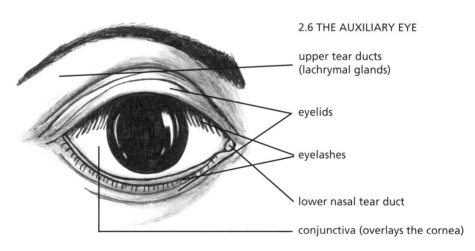

2.6 THE AUXILIARY EYE

upper tear ducts
(lachrymal glands)

eyelids

eyelashes

lower nasal tear duct

conjunctiva (overlays the cornea)

2.7 TWO DIMENSIONAL CROSS-SECTION OF THE EYE

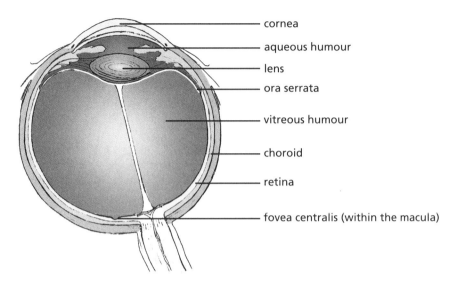

cornea
aqueous humour
lens
ora serrata
vitreous humour
choroid
retina
fovea centralis (within the macula)

There are about 137 million photoreceptors in the retina, about 130 million rods and seven million cones — a ratio of about 95 to 5. Surrounding the retina is the layer of the choroid that supplies the retina with blood. The blood flows within the choroid layer forwards to the ciliary process, which is responsible for secretion of the aqueous humour fluid.

The auxiliary, frontal and interior areas of the eye from the tear fluid all the way through to the lens are all responsible for accommodation (the ability to shift from near to far vision). The retina, on the other hand, is a receiver; it turns light into chemical messages which are transferred into nerve impulses that go to the brain.

Pathways into the brain

From the retina information passes as nerve impulses through the optic nerves (with their partial crossover at the chiasm) around the brainstem to the lateral geniculate bodies of the thalamus (see figures 2.8 & 2.9). Information from the fovea centralis for high resolution or focused seeing and colour perception passing through fibres (the visual radiation, or what I call the lower visual radiation) to the visual cortex, traditionally called the striate cortex or primary visual cortex. I call this the lower visual cortex. This is the part of the visual brain responsible for focused vision and colour perception. I refer to this whole route as the lower visual pathway — the pathway for clear sight.

2.8 LOWER VISUAL PATHWAYS

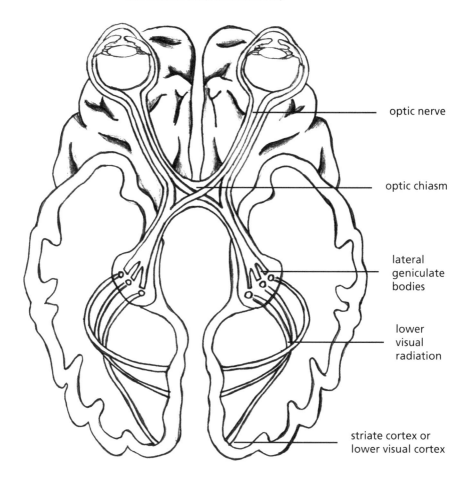

optic nerve

optic chiasm

lateral geniculate bodies

lower visual radiation

striate cortex or lower visual cortex

How seeing clearly works — the conventional view

To see clearly, light needs to be focused not only by the lens, but also by the cornea, in addition to being somewhat refracted by both the tear fluid and the aqueous humour and perhaps even the vitreous humour, before it gets to the fovea centralis. Messages go from here via the optic nerve pathways to the lateral geniculate bodies and on (via fibres of the visual radiation) to the lower visual cortex.

If eyesight is blurry and we need glasses, the commonly held view is that the eye has changed its shape (see figure 2.10). For example, in the case of near- or short-sightedness (myopia), the conventional view is that because the eyeball is elongated, light is focused before it reaches the fovea centralis. The brain then perceives a blur in the distance. A pair

31

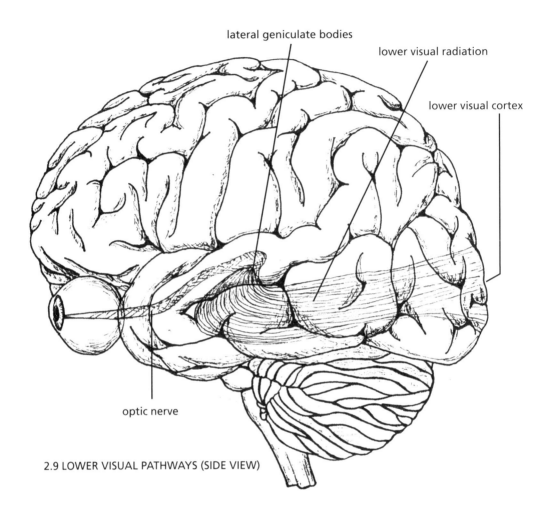

lateral geniculate bodies

lower visual radiation

lower visual cortex

optic nerve

2.9 LOWER VISUAL PATHWAYS (SIDE VIEW)

of concave lenses (see figure 2.11) — the traditional tool for seeing clearly — is cut in such a way that the light is bent to 'hit' the fovea centralis, and the brain perceives clarity.

In the case of long- or far-sightedness from an early age (hyper-metropia), the eyeball is too wide, thus shortening the whole eye (see figure 2.10). Sometimes it is believed that the eyeball is too small. Convex lenses are cut so that once again the light 'hits' the fovea centralis (see figure 2.11). The brain now clearly perceives objects close up which were formerly blurred.

Are there other possibilities?

It is commonly thought that the eyes and the visual system function only as a tool for seeing — and the clearer the seeing the better. Glasses, contact lenses and lately laser surgery reinforce this notion and are used all over the world to facilitate clear eyesight. But might there be long-term side effects from wearing glasses or having surgery? Do the eyes and the visual system have a greater purpose than eyesight?

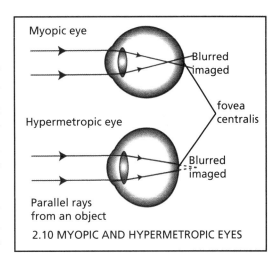

2.10 MYOPIC AND HYPERMETROPIC EYES

Eye-body discoveries

As I mentioned in the Introduction, in 1992, about a year after completely letting go of my glasses I was sitting one day in my studio in Auckland, New Zealand. I was pondering my astigmatism, an irregular curvature of the cornea, which I had had since childhood. I wondered if it was possible to access my corneas and I started to think about them, especially about their insides. As I did this I got a kinaesthetic sense of them. When the thought of tightening my corneas went through my mind I noticed a marked slumping in my chest area.

As an Alexander teacher it would have been easy for me to rectify this and to move out of my slump. Instead I stayed with it, but this time I directed my corneas to release. Instantly my chest moved out of the slump into uprightness.

Now very curious, I again 'went inside' my corneas; when I thought of tightening the corneas the same process of slumping happened in my chest area. Like a yo-yo my body went up and down, just as a result of my thinking into my corneas. Intrigued, I wanted to find out more.

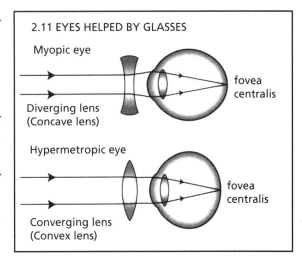

During the following weeks I asked some of my students if they too could direct their corneas. They could, and to my amazement the chest tightening and releasing happened for them too, without fail. What was this connection between the corneas and the chest?

A turning point

I did not know at that time that this was a turning point to an entirely different way of working practically with eyesight, posture, emotions and even functions of the brain — simultaneously and naturally.

As I had been short-sighted I knew my eyeball was elongated, and therefore my retina too. My next question was about the retina: was there any part of the body relating to the retina? There was indeed… by thinking into my retinas, as I had my corneas, I noticed my lower back started to change from tightening to releasing. I became taller and more balanced over my pelvis.

Over the following months I continued to discover relationships between different parts of my eyes and particular areas of the body. Was it just me? No. Experiments with my students showed consistent relationships. When I put down some of these relationships on paper, I discovered a systematic patterning of the eye and the body. I called these the Eye-Body Reflex Patterns. (Over the years my understanding of these relationships has grown and deepened and in the back of this book you will find a map which reflects my current understanding.)

Eye-Body Reflex Patterns: the overview

As I continued to investigate I discovered a full body map relating not only to the eyes but also to the entire visual system. Like the meridians in Chinese medicine or hand and foot reflexology, these are relationships that occur universally, and it is clear to me now that the brain is an integral part of this system.

The eyelids and the layer of conjunctiva are associated with the head and the neck region; the eyeball itself (from the cornea to the entrance of the optic nerve) is associated with the torso; the extrinsic part of the eye (the sclera) and the entire outer sheath of the optic nerves reflect the arms and hands; the visual pathways such as the optic nerves and the visual radiation represent the legs; and the visual cortex the feet (see colour foldout map on the back of this book).

If we see it from the perspective of the body, the head and neck correspond with the eyelids and conjunctiva, the torso with the eyeball, the hands and arms with the sclera and outer sheath of the optic nerves, the upper and lower legs with the optic nerves, and the feet with the visual cortex.

If the eyeball and therefore the retina is elongated, then the lower back will be correspondingly affected. If we are kicked in the shin and a bruise appears, this will be reflected in the visual pathway as well. It's as if the eyes and the whole process of seeing are a microcosm of the body. They are completely interrelated in specific ways.

Experiential anatomy and physiology

By experimenting with my own vision I have been able to identify the general Eyebody Patterns and pathways to the brain. I have devised specific processes to make contact with different areas of the visual system which I frequently use in my group and individual teachings. With this growing understanding of my own visual system I am able to guide people step-by-step through the process of regaining the ability to use their own visual system efficiently.

The higher visual system functions: coordination and integration

I have described the pathway of the cones in the retina via the fovea centralis into the lower visual cortex (the area for the brain for clear sight). Less is known about the pathway for the rods — 95% of the photoreceptors in our retinas. It is clear to me that this pathway is responsible for much more than eyesight. It has tremendous potential for the integration of healthy bodies, clear thinking, emotional balance, spiritual connectedness and lively yet coordinated brain functioning, as well as the ability to manifest change in the physiology of the visual pathways.

The lateral geniculate bodies (part of the thalamus) are an important crossroads. The fovea information from the cones travels through here, then goes straight to the lower visual cortex to provide clear sight. The other 95% of photoreceptors, the rods, which are used for peripheral vision — what I call panoramic vision — travel forward and up from the lateral geniculate bodies through the thalamus, alongside the pineal gland to the third ventricle. Some information continues from here forward to the hypothalamus and pituitary gland (see figure 2.12).

Let me very simply illustrate this. As you read these words, you are probably using your focused vision. Focus intently on these words. Now, change direction; use your panoramic vision, allowing your thoughts to widen the retina and choroid, and still see the page. You may notice that things look different; you may even notice a change in your breathing or how you feel. When you think of using your panoramic vision you are accessing, by means of your intention, more of your rod receptors and thereby stimulating different pathways in your brain. In Chapter 8 you will find detailed instructions to help you use panoramic vision.

Using panoramic vision actually stimulates the functions of the thalamus and hypothalamus, essential for the optimal functioning of the entire physical mechanism. If the thalamus and hypothalamus are not being adequately stimulated by panoramic vision, the parasympathetic functions of the body — such as the heartbeat and breathing — will suffer and the body will be adversely affected. This happens when we use focused vision exclusively; we stimulate only the lower visual pathway.

From the lateral geniculate bodies forward and up through the thalamus and posterior to the third ventricle, information from the rods passes through the limbic system (the emotional brain) and what I call the upper visual radiation to the upper region of the visual cortex, or as I call it, the upper visual cortex. The region back and up from the third ventricle through the limbic system into the upper visual cortex is what

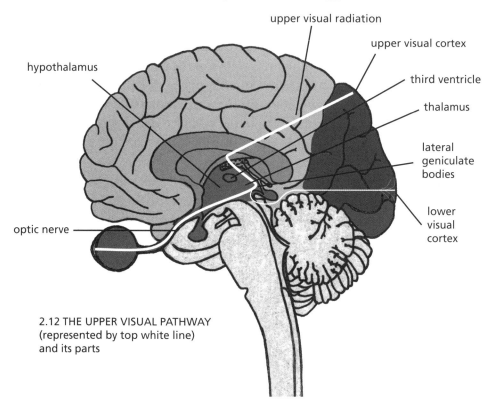

2.12 THE UPPER VISUAL PATHWAY
(represented by top white line)
and its parts

I call the upper visual radiation. What I refer to as the upper visual cortex is situated behind and above the thalamus and limbic system, behind and above the corpus callosum, in the occipito-parietal lobe, above the lower visual cortex. This route is what I call the upper visual pathway.

The brain's connection to the Eyebody Patterns

Years after I discovered the first Eyebody connections I became aware of further relationships between the visual system and the eyes, building on what I already understood. Here is an outline of the connections between the various parts of the brain (reptilian, limbic and neocortex) and the eyes: the thalamus relates to the interior parts of the eye; the limbic brain relates to the anterior part of the eye; the upper part of the neocortex (upper visual cortex) relates to the auxiliary parts of the eye. I continue to refer to this entire system as the Eyebody Patterns, even though I now understand that these patterns arise out of the brain (see foldout map of Eyebody Patterns, inside back cover).

Departing from the conventional view

The conventional view is that the eye itself is the presenting problem; as I see it, this is merely a symptom. Glasses, contact lenses and refractive surgery address only this symptom, to the detriment of the visual system overall as well as the physical, mental and emotional well-being of their recipient. By addressing the effect rather than the ultimate cause, our natural vision is not able to emerge and the multiple functions of the visual system — other than clear eyesight — are inhibited. My understanding is that all visual dysfunction arises not in the eyes themselves, but in the brain; specifically in the function of the upper visual cortex. The upper visual cortex guides the whole visual system.

The upper visual cortex has the potential to integrate the entire visual system by means of what I call conscious depth perception. Conscious depth perception is a mental direction (akin to panoramic vision), which creates coordination and integration of all regions of the brain. Through this mechanism a dynamic balance is achieved within the entire system that results in clarity of sight and thinking alike.

*

In the next chapter we will discover more about the multiple functions of the visual system and look at the primary coordinating mechanism — and how this affects the brain, eyes and body.

3

Fundamental types of visual brain function

Primary and secondary functions

As mentioned in the last chapter, the visual system has multiple functions — it does much more than just see. There are two levels of visual system function. The primary function is the coordination of our physical, emotional and mental states. Primary functions are what we need for basic coordination and optimal functioning to keep us going, keep us alive — physically, emotionally and mentally. The visual system and pathways are present in each of our three brains: reptilian, limbic and neocortex. This is why the visual system is so fundamental. It needs to be working well so we can breathe, digest our food, move around, make appropriate decisions or sleep at night — optimally. Because of our inborn resilience, we are able to function without our primary functions working perfectly, but often just to a point.

Clear sight is a secondary function of the visual system. Secondary functions are more external, such as reading, computing, looking for our keys, or communicating with others — and seeing clearly when we need to. This may be surprising, so I will restate it: *clear sight is a secondary, not a primary, function of the visual system*. These secondary functions can only work well when the primary functions are in order. For most of us the primary functions are strongly compromised — perhaps without our knowledge. This means the secondary functions (the activities of daily life) become exhausting and full of effort. We begin to try harder to do things right. Life becomes hard work.

New pathways can be created within the brain so that we can harmonize the primary functions, thus enabling us to perform the secondary functions effortlessly. The whole body, including the brain, then has the ability to work to its full potential. Our emotional and spiritual self will be affected by this new coordination as well, with an increased feeling of safety, satisfaction and overall well-being.

The upper visual cortex: two distinctive types

Major differences in the upper visual cortex — whether it is overextended or contracted — appear to underlie two parallel distinctive types (see figure 3.1). We seem to be born with either one of these predominant patterns within our upper visual cortex. I am not certain when exactly the upper visual cortex type manifests itself, but I would think well before birth — perhaps around the time of conception. It appears to me that the upper visual cortex type is neither acquired through experience nor changes from one type to another — rather, it is an inborn characteristic. Because the upper visual cortex guides our visual system these distinctive differences lead us to different visual experiences, internally and externally, and may ultimately result in hypermetropia, myopia or any other visual dysfunction.

To simplify and put things in a practical context, the overextended visual cortex underlies hypermetropia (long- or far-sightedness from an early age), and the contracted upper visual cortex underlies myopia (near- or short-sightedness). Myopia and hypermetropia are two of the most prominent visual dysfunctions, but all others (astigmatism, presbyopia, glaucoma, cataracts, crossed-eyes, etc.) result from and develop out of one of these two distinctive upper visual cortex types as well. Even with clear sight these types are part of us and may at some point in life contribute to visual dysfunction whether or not we are aware of it.

The overextended upper visual cortex

People with this pattern see everything rather big — often bigger than life. Any thought pattern, any idea, any project is much bigger than that which contracted type people might conceive. Many people with this pattern report a tendency to 'woosh out' — that is to disconnect from the self and the environment.

About 10 to 20 percent of the population seem to fall into this category. They stand out, they are different. In a world of predominantly contracted upper visual cortexes they somehow don't fit in. Their world is much larger and they are often misunderstood. Their visual cortex works in such a way that it is over-widened. Pressure results from the over-widening (and from seeing the visual pathways as so large) which directly affects the lens and the entire front area of the eye. This can lead to frustration and a short temper, especially when dealing with those 'small' brains of the opposite character type. The overextended character type seems to have little patience for how others think. Grandiosity and ambition are also characteristic. Everything seen so clearly in the distance is to be strived for. Nothing less than fabulous will do. This again can cause loads of frustration, as sometimes small, step-by-step processes might be needed to achieve a goal.

Because of the over-widening, the close-up world becomes threatening and letting people in can be a challenge. They tend to keep people away and hide their fear by being strong and sometimes overpowering. There may sometimes be a sense of aloofness when they are dealing with the opposite type. Their emotional boundaries are very strong, even rigid, and it takes a sense of safety and trust to overcome the fear of letting anything come too close. In children this mechanism often doesn't allow for close bonds.

Although they feel more strained and overfocused dealing with details close-up (which lets part of their visual system switch off) overextended types are brilliant organizers. Along with this comes a sense of vigilance. There may be very clear distance sight and also very keen hearing. There may be a hyper-awareness of sounds, as a way of keeping tabs on what's happening around them. It can feel overwhelming to have so much information coming in, bombarding them.

The overextended world is not an easy one. Seeing and experiencing everything so big, the 'small world' of the other 80 to 90 percent somehow doesn't make much sense. Why be so small when you can be big?

This overextended type underlies hypermetropia (also known as long- or far-sightedness, starting at an early age), often crossed-eyes, sometimes presbyopia or glaucoma and in some cases cataracts and sensitivity to light. Some people with clear sight might be of this type. If glasses are prescribed, perhaps for hypermetropia, letting go of wearing them is usually quite easy, as they may only be needed for reading. Glasses may be worn for security when in emotionally close-up situations. Once overextended character types recognize this, the glasses can stay off.

From an Eyebody Pattern perspective, the overextended pattern leads to an over-widened visual pathway throughout the neocortex, limbic system and reptilian brain which leads to an over-widening of the eye. In particular, the parts of the front of the eye — the pupil, iris, aqueous humour fluid, canal of Schlemm, cornea and the eyelids — are overly wide. Physically, this manifests as tension held within the bone structure of the skull, the neck and shoulder areas, the breathing and especially the heart. All of these are affected.

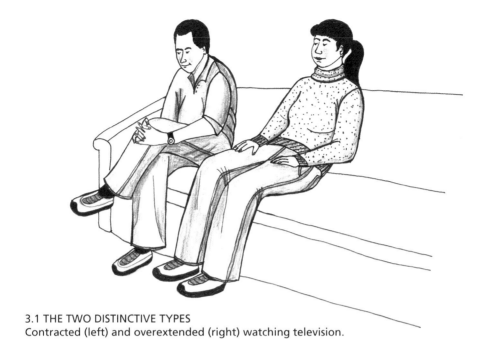

3.1 THE TWO DISTINCTIVE TYPES
Contracted (left) and overextended (right) watching television.

Once overextended types start integrating their visual system they generally reap tremendous benefits. They start connecting more easily with people, and their frustrations with self and others transform into enjoyment. They see clearly up close and in the distance with ease — and have a sense of living life more fully.

The contracted upper visual cortex

The majority of people, between 80 and 90 percent, will find themselves relating to this type. This type rules our modern world.

The contracted character type has a detailed mind, accurate at times, but woozy at others. There is a tendency to narrowly focus in life, to see the small picture. The contracted upper visual cortex type has the potential to develop myopia (near- or short-sightedness) and to see really small details close-up very clearly — even if presbyopia (middle-age vision) develops, the mental tendency is still present though close-up eyesight becomes blurry.

Mentally, this character type is associated with frontal lobe thinking, over-focusing on detail and generally a lack of overall vision or larger perspective. Here the tendency is to mind-wander, to dwell on old memories and get stuck there. This detracts from the ability to be in the moment.

Emotionally, the underlying pattern relates to fear, anxiety, frustration, lack of self-esteem and a narrowing uptightness. The general disposition is friendly.

From an Eyebody perspective, the upper visual cortex qualitatively spirals forwards and down, affecting the auxiliary area of the eye. The limbic brain is then caused to press forward, thus contracting the frontal areas of the eye and changing its shape. As a result of this frontal contraction the pupil, retina, choroid and vitreous humour will also tighten, resulting in non-stimulation of the thalamus, as information from the peripheral photoreceptors of the retina are not receiving enough light. This lack of stimulation will narrow the thalamus, moving it backwards and down. The resulting tightening of the optic nerves will pull the eyeball back into an elongating shape. This means the retina cannot carry out its panoramic functions and the fovea centralis will be overworking. With the thalamus not getting enough stimuli, there is a resulting shortening of the brainstem that brings about a slumping in the body. This is the pattern of myopia. The whole coordinating process of the primary functions of the visual system is hampered. Here we find the upper visual cortex not being used to its full potential.

The contracted character type's body posture is often stooped with the head and brainstem tilting back and downward. The lower back, pelvis and upper legs to the knees are especially affected.

The body may show signs of overstrain in the liver, spleen and kidneys, difficulty in respiration and digestion, sometime headaches or migraines and there may be reproductive dysfunctions later in life.

Contracted character types may develop myopia in early childhood or up to about age 21 and/or presbyopia from age 40-45. Even people with good eyesight might be in this category. Other dysfunctions originating from the contracted upper visual cortex type are cataracts, glaucoma, astigmatism, floaters and more.

In contracted types the limbic system, where we store old memories, needs the weight lifted off it. By learning to integrate the limbic aspect of the visual system, contracted character types can experience more harmony. Without needing to name or rehash any of our old stories, the memory bank can be cleared and cleansed as things are let go. Simultaneously, the integrating process leads to better body function and an enlivening of the entire visual system that will help develop a clearer long-term vision for self and surroundings.

A combination of contraction and overextension is possible if you are short-sighted in one eye and long-sighted in the other. This often leads to headaches, tremendous physical tension, and fatigue as both sides of the visual pathway, body and brain, are functioning in opposing manners. But this can integrated.

Cause and effect relating to overextension or contraction

We all have one of these upper visual cortex tendencies. Whether or not a visual dysfunction is present, the functioning of the entire visual system is still affected by one predisposition or the other. Where there is a visual dysfunction, it always seems to come back to what is happening in the upper visual cortex, whether contracted or overextended, which affects the function of the entire visual system. Putting on a pair of glasses or contact lenses or having laser eye surgery deals with the effect but not the cause. For a fundamental change in the visual system we need to address the cause, so the effect will be different. The eyes receive their directions from the upper visual cortex, so for any fundamental vision improvement it is vital that the upper visual cortex be fully engaged.

*

How do we address the cause? In the next chapter we will discover principles which, when applied to the visual system, create the possibility for integration, no matter what the upper visual cortex type. The existence of these fundamental upper visual cortex types is the first principle of this work and the rest are built upon that.

4

The Eyebody Principles

The Oxford English Dictionary defines *principle* as: 'A fundamental truth or proposition … essential to a system of thought…'

Principles are universal constants; they remain true no matter what the circumstances. My work is principle-based.

The Eyebody Principles

1. **Upper visual cortex types:** There are at least two fundamental, inborn types of upper visual cortex function that can only be changed by means of our consciousness. Upper visual cortex types have been discussed at length in the previous chapter.

2. **Brain, eye and body patterns:** The Eyebody Patterns govern the whole self. Within the visual system we find a homunculus of the whole person: the brain, eye, body patterns which include physical, mental, emotional and spiritual facets.

3. **Primary coordinating mechanism:** There is a primary coordinating mechanism housed in the upper visual cortex which is stimulated through the generation of conscious depth perception.

4. **Vision leads**, the eyes, body and environment follow.

Before I discuss the principles in detail, let's look at some issues which surround and underlie them.

Principles versus exercises

The brain is the generator of all activity. Thought itself is a type of activity, visible in MRI scans as an electro-chemical process similar to the brain function that happens during actual movement. In fact, research has shown that actual movement and the mere thought of movement are very nearly the same thing within the brain. Some levels of activity, such as breathing, digestion and circulation, are governed by the autonomic nervous system and are considered to be involuntary. We do not need to think about them to make them happen.

Much of our movement also takes place without our having to think about it. For example, when I walk I do not have to think, 'bend knee, extend leg', etc — my brain has learned a habitual way of taking care of this. My brain coordinates my walking and I don't experience that I've been thinking about the process at all. This can be likened to the pre-set buttons on a car radio — it is not necessary to know the station wavelength or turn the dial left or right: we only have to press a button to get the desired station. The brain is filled with well-worn pathways so that we can perform most of the activities of life without having to think consciously about them.

Conscious thinking is the activity that helps stimulate new pathways in the brain. Our ability as intelligent beings to make conscious choices and decisions, to direct not only our actions but also our intentions and our thoughts, is what underlies this work. When principles are in place we are able to use our brains consciously in a consistent manner.

A word about exercises: I can do them for the rest of my life and fundamentally nothing may change. If they are habitually done I proceed in using my brain in the same old way. The only benefit I may have is to feel virtuous in having done my exercises — and exercises may make me feel good, increase blood flow and get things moving. There is usually no harm in this and there can be many benefits, but when we're looking to make fundamental change, it is *principles* that are critical. Of course, when we apply principles to the activity of doing exercises, the entire activity can be enriched and take on an entirely different quality; the exercise is then secondary to the active application of the principles.

Central to the principles of this work is the understanding that eyesight and vision are flexible; each of us has a habitual way of using our eyes and visual system that can be changed. I am able to constructively influence my visual system and eyesight directly and, by doing so, my body and brain functions indirectly.

Any discussion of the principles underpinning this work needs to acknowledge in particular FM Alexander, the creator of the Alexander Technique. Its principles have helped me greatly on my voyage of discovery. Those of you who are familiar with the Alexander Technique will know that it too is principle-based and you may recognize Alexander's ideas underlying much of my own thinking.

Kinaesthesia and the visual system

Kinaesthesia, our sense of how our own movement feels, is sometimes called our 'lost sixth sense'. It is closely related to proprioception: how I know where my body parts are without having to move them, or even look at them. A reliable kinaesthetic sense is vital to the effective, efficient and well coordinated functioning of the visual system, because it enables me to have a reliable sense of internal reference. This leads to an increased sense of lightness in the eye and the optic nerves, easier 'access' to the fluids within the eye and an internal sense of the reptilian brain, limbic brain and neocortex. It's the mental ability to visually direct our intention that develops this kinaesthetic awareness.

But we cannot afford to rely on kinaesthesia alone as a tool for improving the visual system. Alexander has written in great detail about how our kinaesthetic and proprioceptive senses are very often unreliable. We become so accustomed to our habits that they feel right to us, even if they are interfering with our ability to function naturally. Our present sensory awareness is based on the faulty assumption that we are totally coordinated. Thus we would like to use our kinaesthetic sense as a reference point only, rather than relying on it as a tool.

What am I doing?

If I cannot reliably know what I am doing, how is change possible? I need to learn to stop and figure out what I am doing, to cultivate the ability to observe the process of my own thinking. It is necessary to stop, to listen to my thought process and to look at what I am doing within my visual system. We can, because of our human ability to think consciously, learn to observe objectively what is going on within our visual system and over time understand our visual habits. This is fundamental; otherwise I continue my habitual thinking and my habitual ways of seeing, moving, feeling and behaving. I can first observe my mental activity and second make choices about it — and, if I so choose, improve the quality and efficiency of the visual system. This is fundamental to the process of change. I may hope and hope for change or improvement, but if I am unaware and stay with my old patterns of thinking and behaviour, change is not possible. By cultivating the ability to consciously observe I can discover what I am doing on the inside and create the possibility of change.

Use affects function

If I use my eyes with excessive tension, my body will respond by being excessively tense. If I am in the habit of overly focusing on things, my body will respond by being held and overworked. If I spend my time trying really hard to see things, my brain, eyes and body will all be exhausted.

The way I use my eyes affects how they function. The way I use my visual cortex will affect how my visual cortex functions. The way I use my brain will affect the function of my brain. The way I use my body will affect the function of my body. The way I use my upper visual cortex will affect all of these.

The idea that we *use* ourselves all the time, consciously or unconsciously, and that the quality of that use directly affects the quality of our functioning, is one of the basic tenets of Alexander's work. This means the way we sit and stand, the way we habitually react to emotional situations, the way we think about things, all have direct bearing on the way we move through life.

Our visual system is also subject to this law. The way I engage my visual cortex will have a direct effect on how I see, as well as on how my entire brain and body work.

The visual system, because of its overall coordinating role, multiple functions and inherent subtlety, can undo tension throughout the body. Releasing tension within the visual system needs to be done through the visual system itself. The visual system, as part of the brain, is at the top of the chain of command. The brain, visual system and body are part of an interwoven mechanism. Each part plays its role and it is the coordination of the totality that enables optimum functioning.

The first principle: Fundamental, inborn types of upper visual cortex function

The first principle is that there are at least two fundamental, inborn types of upper visual cortex function that can only be changed by means of our consciousness. The overextended and contracted upper visual cortex types have been discussed at length in the previous chapter. All of the preceding underlies the principles which follow.

The second principle: The Eyebody Patterns govern the whole self

The second principle is that the whole person is governed by the visual system. The Eyebody Patterns are universally present in all of us. That said, I will explain some issues surrounding and underlying these patterns.

Habitually inefficient ways of using the visual system are what cause difficulty with our eyesight, imbalances in our emotions and functional problems in the body. For example, if I habitually tighten my cornea, there will be a resulting problem with my eyesight (perhaps astigmatism), a corresponding difficulty in my interpersonal communications and probably a tightening of my shoulder area as well. This pattern happens whether I am aware of it or not. From my observation any physical, mental or emotional experience at its core arises out of the visual system.

When I direct an area of my visual system, let's say the retina to use its panoramic field of vision, the pelvis and lower back will follow by freeing, perhaps lengthening and widening. If I think of freeing my pelvis and lower back, the retina will not follow — the impulse of widening needs to originate within the visual system.

Let's say I am involved in an accident and I hurt my lower back. Experience tells me that the visual system is also affected — the retina and vitreous humour (in this case) as well as the overall coordinating mechanism of the reptilian brain and limbic system and the neocortex. This may not be apparent unless there is a change from clear sight to blurriness. The pain may go away, whether over time or by means of physical intervention, but the contraction, pain or trauma of the lower back can still be found in the visual system, even years later, whether or not I am aware of it. Because of the resulting imbalance, more visual habits can form over the long haul that will affect the entire visual system, in some cases leading to eyesight problems.

If I have sessions of cranial osteopathy, Feldenkrais, Alexander, structural integration, massage, physiotherapy, chiropractic, or other body or mind/body work, my body may feel lighter and I may feel more aware and alive, and pain-free. I might be thinking more clearly, be more coordinated and in better shape. But this is likely to have only a marginal affect on my visual system as the appropriate relationship of the brain region to the eye area has not been addressed directly. Only when we bring consciousness into the visual system can these patterns be dissolved from the source. To make fundamental changes in the visual system, it needs to be addressed directly. Discovery of the visual pathway, learning the mental processes for accessing the upper visual cortex and applying conscious depth perception (which are discussed later in this chapter) while making contact with the environment, creates fundamental change in the different layers of the brain, resulting in complete psycho-physical integration.

There are other systems in which one part of the body governs all other parts of the body — Chinese medicine, for example, relates to the entire body through the meridian system. Hand, foot or ear reflexology addresses the whole body through the hand, foot or ear, with specific areas corresponding to each area of the human body.

The Eyebody Patterns differ from these other systems in several ways. Because the visual system is part of the brain, it exists at a more fundamental level of our organization. Brain tissue is the source of our movement and physicality; the foot, to use reflexology as an example, while it may indeed relate with other parts of the system, is itself still governed by the brain, first and foremost. Any homunculus existing outside the brain is, by its very nature, secondary. In addition, the Eyebody Patterns depend upon conscious visualization as a tool, rather than anything purely mechanical. When I use the brain itself as a tool for change, the change cannot help but be more fundamental and more lasting than anything that originates in a peripheral part of the body. By using our ability to make conscious decisions we are able to make truly lasting change.

Multiple functions of the visual system: physical, emotional, mental, spiritual, and interaction with the environment

When I first discovered the relationship between the eyes and the body I thought that was it. Then I noticed the visual pathways leading into the thalamus, which coordinates sensory information coming from the body. From there I noticed the visual pathway passing through the limbic system and began to understand its relationship with the frontal area of the eye. Here I found a relationship to the old memories stored and held deep inside our brain — and the visual system's role therein. The apex is the upper visual cortex, which relates to the auxiliary part of the eye. The upper visual cortex is the seat of consciously directed depth perception, which integrates the entire visual pathway from the brain areas to the eye and beyond, allowing for the synthesis of self with environment.

Each layer of the brain has a specific overall relationship to the visual system: the reptilian brain relates to the physical function of the body, the limbic system relates to the emotional functions and the neocortex to the mental functions. Conscious depth perception, as the integration and coordination of all, relates to a finer, beyond the physical, spiritual function. This conscious depth perception integrates not only the functions of the brain and eyes, but extends itself to the environment, surrounding objects, the contact with the outside world.

The third principle: The primary coordinating mechanism

FM Alexander wrote of a 'primary control mechanism' which he said coordinates the movement of the whole body. He specified that this mechanism must be operating for the whole self to function properly. He understood this to be the head-neck-back relationship. My experience is that a deeper mechanism lies within the brain.

The third principle is that there is a primary coordinating mechanism situated in the upper visual cortex which is stimulated by the generation of conscious depth perception. This coordinates the multiple functions of the visual system and therefore the whole self. It integrates the visual pathway through the neocortex, limbic system and reptilian brain and coordinates the whole. This coordination includes, among other things, the thalamus and hypothalamus, which in turn coordinate our senses, heartbeat, breathing, hormonal balance and many other involuntary processes, and allows for the optimal functioning of the whole system. In other words, conscious depth perception is an overall link to and for our whole brain — coordinating our whole self without our having to think of the parts directly.

We often speak of things being 'in depth' or 'deep.' When describing a person, a school of thought, an artwork or the like, depth is a certain quality that we understand. Perhaps we don't know how to get to it or create it, but we know it when we see it. Something with depth has multiple layers or functions and perhaps a sense of profundity or universality. By the same token, 'shallow' has negative connotations. It is possible to consciously access my own depth, to integrate all of my own functions and facets and be fully present with myself and others by applying this conscious depth perception. Many artists, writers, yogi and spiritual seekers have come up with various means like meditation or drugs to achieve a similar experience. I have found that the key to getting there is conscious depth perception from the upper visual cortex. This also happens to be the same means to achieve clear sight and ease in all the other secondary functions of the visual system.

The integration produced by conscious depth perception includes seeing clearly and sharply, distinguishing light and darkness, colour, movement, depth and forms or shapes; it also includes emotional behaviour and responses, along with facets of communication with the external world and spiritual aspects of oneness. All have their respective area in the brain and in the visual pathways, with correlating physical responses; conscious depth perception brings them together as a unified, optimally-functioning whole.

If the visual pathways in their entirety are not being stimulated properly (or not at all) my overall functioning will be impaired whether I am aware of it or not, resulting in poor eyesight, pain, inability to think clearly, disconnection from self or others, and other maladies, general or specific.

With practice the process of specifically stimulating my brain in this way gradually allows my overall functioning to become more efficient and effortless and optimises my well-being.

This primary coordinating mechanism integrates and enlivens the operation of the neocortex for clearer abstract thinking, decision making and visualizing; integrates the limbic system, giving an effect of emotional lightness and freedom; and affects the reptilian brain with its thalamus and hypothalamus, improving physical coordination, ease of movement and functioning — and the eyes follow as well.

Conscious depth perception

By now you are probably wondering what this tremendous integrator is. Conscious depth perception is an internal thinking/visualizing process by which I visualize from the upper visual cortex panoramic space within the depth of the retinas (for contracted types), then bring attentiveness from the lower visual cortex to beneath the surface of an object.

Conscious depth perception happens within the upper quadrant of the visual cortex. It automatically, consistently and reliably initiates a process that frees the entire visual system and body. It is the absolute primary mechanism which coordinates the visual pathway, body, nervous system and the brain's thinking processes simultaneously.

During my workshops I ask participants to place their hands on the back of my skull to illustrate from the outside what can happen when this primary coordinating mechanism is activated. When I use my conscious depth perception the person with his or her hands on my head usually says something like, "I can feel your skull moving slightly", "Your brain here seems to have more activity", "The bones are moving," or "It feels everything is expanding further back and your whole head is more balanced on top of your spine."

Conscious depth perception activates new brain pathways. This in turn creates a new freedom towards the front. The neocortex is then able to lighten up off the reptilian brain, allowing the entire brainstem to be less contracted, or in the case of the overextended pattern, to be more coordinated. The nervous system and the entire body can then function with increased freedom. At the same time, subtle pressure can be released from the eyes so that they can function more effectively. The frontal lobes and the auditory area of the brain (located beneath the diencephalon) can function more easily without pressure from above. This results in clearer thinking and better hearing.

The fourth principle: Vision leads

Bennis and Nanus (1985) describe vision as: "A mental image of a possible and desirable future state of the organism … as vague as a dream or as precise as a goal or mission statement … a view of a realistic, credible, attractive future for the organization, a condition that is better in some important ways than what now exists."

I like to define vision holistically as the interaction of the coordinated visual system (which, of course, includes the whole person in depth) with the environment, including the goal, the new organization, and the desired outcomes, such as reading and understanding the book in my hands right now, or whatever my desire might be.

The fourth principle is that vision leads and eyes, body, and environment follow. The upper visual cortex leads by means of conscious depth perception and the rest of the brain, eyes, and body follow when we make contact in depth with the surrounding environment.

The higher functions of the visual system lead the whole person — and guide our contact with external surroundings as well; the people around us, the situations we find ourselves in, and the choices we make. Earlier I mentioned that vision is really our primary sense; only the visual system so comprehensively exists and travels through all the layers of the brain. No other sense or system does this.

In modern society the frontal lobes tend to dominate. The result of this from a vision perspective is that the lower visual cortex overworks and the upper visual cortex stagnates. This leads to a disconnection from our selves and others that is nearly a hallmark of contemporary society. The way we live has become increasingly disconnected — from our selves, what we really want in life and what we are able to envision in the future. The decisions we in modern society are making in many arenas are generally short-sighted — an overall vision is lacking.

How do I change? The first step is to coordinate my entire visual system, so that its multiple functions can operate efficiently and effectively. This first step makes sure that I as a human being am coordinated and functioning optimally. Then I can apply this primary visual function to desired outcomes — all from within the upper visual cortex, coordinated by conscious depth perception. My brain, eyes and body are then following my desired outcome with ease and efficiency — and the resulting continuity between my self and my environment ensures that the whole follows suit.

As Galen Cranz says in the foreword to this book, there is a philosophical concept called 'emergence' in which the future shapes the past, the envisioned shapes our present. When I visualize in depth in the way I have described, the whole is more powerful than the sum of its parts. Vision leading means that my internal coordination and my external environment are continuous — as I harmonize my internal vision it is incorporated into my surroundings. The internal and the external can be merged synergistically by coordinating the higher functions of the brain.

Visualizing from the frontal area of the neocortex does not have the same powerful effects; in fact it creates two-dimensional outcomes. This sort of visualisation has not activated the pathways of the visual system — overall coordination is lacking and therefore excludes the limbic system for memory and emotional balance and the reptilian brain for coordinating our physicality with our intention. For these reasons this frontal lobe visualizing may not bring you the outcomes you desire.

If I habitually bypass my visual pathway I will be without the primary coordinating mechanism, lacking the appropriate vision necessary to guide me efficiently through life. As I see it, this is one reason so many of us experience pain and discomfort in our lives, physically, mentally and emotionally.

When the body or emotions are all I have to lead me I can feel disconnected, leaderless. The intellectual, factual mind may dominate, but this lacks integration. Without vision generated within the upper visual cortex leading, the body and emotions do their thing without clear guidance. This is surviving rather than thriving.

The frontal lobes do not coordinate the whole as vision generated within the upper visual cortex does. We place a high value on frontal lobe thinking in modern culture. Our frontal lobes are able to deliver information, news, facts and statistics. These are all important currencies in the modern world. The work most of us do at computers — some of us all day, every day — is possible because of our frontal lobes. But it's safe to say that no one experiences a heightened sense of coordination and wholeness after a day at the computer. Our frontal lobes are sophisticated and important, but they do not coordinate our whole selves.

True vision includes the primary coordination of brain, eyes and body and it extends itself to the world around us, including the outcomes we desire. When our three-dimensional vision leads us, eyes, body and the environment follow harmoniously.

*

In the next chapter we will look at the method itself and how various visual dysfunctions, along with their analogous physical, mental and emotional components, can be changed through the application of these principles.

5

The Eyebody Method and case histories

So far we have explored the anatomy of the eye, my discoveries of the Eyebody Patterns and some of the physiology of the visual system — including the connections of areas of the brain to the body and posture. In the previous chapter we discussed the key principles and ideas that underlie the Eyebody Method.

Central to this is the understanding that eyesight and vision are flexible: each of us has established habits around our eyes, our visual system and our thinking that can be changed. By applying principles and directing our intentions (mentally guiding the visual system) specifically from within we constructively influence our visual system and brain directly, as well as our posture, body and eyesight indirectly.

The Eyebody Patterns — a reliable tool

Every visual dysfunction (such as myopia, presbyopia, astigmatism, glaucoma, cataracts, light sensitivity, eyestrain) is evident as a physical pattern in the visual system, and is accompanied by mental, emotional and physical patterns in the layers of the brain. All these patterns can be changed so that eyesight, brain and body functions can improve.

The presenting problem could be a visual or eye dysfunction (for which glasses or medication may have been prescribed), a specific physical problem (back pain, digestive or breathing problems, for example), or an overall sense that our general health and well-being are not what they could be. The Eyebody Patterns help us get to the root of the problem so that real change is possible. If we focus just on the presenting problems we may keep chasing the moving target of symptoms indefinitely.

Working with a heightened kinaesthetic sense of my own visual system, I am reliably able to determine the state of the visual system (as well as related body and brain function) of the person with whom I am working. I then help to guide the person through their own visual pathway. The guidance includes verbal, visual and tactile communication, all informed by an increasingly clear sense of my own visual system. If an area is not functioning well there is a sense of contraction and lack of coordination. I can then work together with a person to undo this contraction, improving his or her own kinaesthetic sense and thus changing overall functioning and coordination. It becomes easier with practice for students of this method to perceive their inside anatomy and let go of their habits.

The next step is to re-educate and coordinate the visual brain function so that the eyes and the appropriate areas of the brain are 'connected'. People often notice simultaneous changes in body posture and function. Repetition ensures that habits gradually change so that the entire system — brain, eye and body — can function optimally.

Application of the principles to daily activities such as reading, writing, or driving a car is addressed at length in Chapter 7.

As they go through this process, students of the method grow in understanding and experience many visual, physical, emotional and mental changes. In many ways learning this work is like learning a musical instrument. When I first pick up an instrument I have no idea how to play it. With skilled guidance and regular practice I can learn step-by-step how to use the instrument, then gradually to make music at a more and more sophisticated level. With continuing practice I continue the learning process and my understanding becomes increasingly refined. The process is the same in vision work: as I become progressively skilled at working with my visual system I begin to perceive the workings of my brain more clearly and this in turn affects my whole body. In the beginning skilled guidance is needed, but as the practice becomes part of daily life, you make progress towards your goal and can continue on your own.

Visual directions

Appropriate visual directions (which I am continuously developing) set the eyes, optic nerves and brainstem free and allow information to flow freely within the entire visual system. Appropriate visual directions are vital to overextended and contracted upper visual cortex types alike. Mental direction is how this work works. The specific visual directions differ for each upper visual cortex type.

These directions are based on the Eyebody Patterns that are rooted in the anatomy of the visual system — specifically the anatomy of the intrinsic and extrinsic areas of the eyes, visual pathways and areas of the brain.

An example of these visual directions for the contracted type would be first to mentally engage with the peripheral space within your retina (panoramic vision) then to include the choroid layer surrounding the retina, with the intention of your vitreous humour making contact with the expanding retina. This process needs repetition to be learned. With repetition comes new brain pathways. Once the individual parts of the visual system are stimulated, conscious depth perception is added to integrate the parts into a fully functioning whole.

Conscious depth perception is the fundamental ingredient; it is the primary coordinator of the visual system and itself a visual direction. It is the creator of simultaneous change in eyesight, the visual pathways, the nervous system and the body, and the three brains, as well as the finer spiritual planes of the visual system and overall vision. Visual directions are necessary to undo tensions in the visual system, allowing new eye-body coordination to happen. Specific visual directions plus conscious depth perception form the process of re-educating the visual system and its multiple functions.

Real change is challenging. Habits can be difficult to shift. People give up smoking and take it up again; they lose weight and regain it; fall into the familiar slump. When new pathways are not being stimulated in the brain the body continues to get the same old messages, even when the person really wants to change. Nothing will change as long as only the old neural pathways are being trodden. Learning to become aware of where you are in your visual system, to direct your intention and use conscious depth perception makes fundamental change possible.

Glasses and contact lenses: Are there side effects?

Wearing glasses, whether for myopia, presbyopia, hypermetropia or astigmatism, helps to create clear images. But there are also far-reaching side effects. As we have seen, lenses are cut in such a way that light is directed to the fovea centralis, so that the 5% of the brain within the lower visual cortex receives constant, intensive amounts of stimulus and picks up a clear image. A major side effect is that we are using only 5% of the photoreceptors actively and 95% lie dormant. The rest of the retina is not stimulated. And just as the retina is not being stimulated, so the rest of the visual cortex is not being stimulated or activated. A large portion of our brain is being starved of information and stimulation.

Wearing glasses or contact lenses can create patterns of thinking and seeing which may affect the memory and the ability to visualize, while causing an overall subtle contraction of the surrounding bone structures of the skull. Glasses sometimes subdue headaches, although the pattern of headaches will still be present, just below our level of awareness.

It is increasingly common for eye specialists to recommend different corrective lens prescriptions in each eye — one for close and one for far vision — so that there is no need for either reading glasses or bifocals. This affects both visual pathways differently and creates an imbalance in brain function, leading to asymmetry within the visual pathway and the body. It can also lead to mental confusion as the lower visual cortex has to work extra hard to make sense of the information it is getting. This would also be true when refractive surgery is performed to correct one eye for near vision and the other for far vision.

Even while driving, glasses or contact lenses may hinder as well as support us because our peripheral vision is reduced and our attention only goes to the point of clear sightedness. While playing sport glasses may hinder our ability to move in a coordinated way. Glasses or even contact lenses may operate as a barrier to meaningful and open communication with others; inhibiting our ability to naturally see what is in front of us and allow ourselves to be seen.

5.1 "Do I really need glasses for this?"

Friday afternoon glasses

I have had a heavy week. Emotionally I feel lousy, my back hurts and my neck is stiff. My colleague at work went off sick and I had more to do than I could cope with, my children are demanding too much of me, my wife wants me to do more gardening, the weather is wet and grey and in general I feel drowsy. Not to mention my blurry vision. I make an appointment late on Friday afternoon, after all this, with an optometrist. I am rushed and late, but I get there. Sure enough, I need a pair of glasses so I can see clearly again and I get fitted for a pair. Well, somehow things change over the weekend: the weather improves and suddenly springtime is here, beautiful, sunny and dry. It's actually fun and enjoyable to do the garden; I feel emotionally much better; my spirits are raised; there is no more neck and back pain; my boss calls me and says my colleague will be back on Monday and I can take a day off; my children are much happier to have a dad around. All in all my stress levels are greatly reduced. I go and pick up my glasses and wear them every day as I was told, so my brain will get used to them, and indeed it does. But it is likely that with my stress lessened I do not need to use those glasses at all. The thing with glasses is that they override every intention to use panoramic vision. The glasses do the focusing for us and we lose the ability to do so in a natural way. What we don't use, we lose! Often stronger and stronger lenses are prescribed. Our ability to use our brain and the eye in all its subtlety is lost. The side effects may stiffen our bodies, fatigue our eyes and reduce our ability to think clearly, all without addressing the root of the problem.

Refractive surgery

For some years now refractive laser eye surgery has been a big hit. But what are the long-term effects on the eyes, brain, body and emotions? Some people swear by laser surgery: "It takes only a few minutes and costs nothing because my health insurance pays for it!"; "I can see clearly without any glasses, and it took only a few minutes". Yes, most people do see more clearly after the operation and no longer need to wear glasses. However, others suffer from after-effects when the operation does not work out as they had hoped. The most common procedure at this time is for the frontal layer of the cornea to be folded open, with the second layer 'scraped off' so that the maximum light reaches the fovea centralis, just as with glasses. The first layer heals relatively quickly and 'seals' the second layer of the cornea again. This 'scraping off' is permanent. I find people often complain that they have not achieved the desired results: they may still have to use glasses (though less strong), or have difficulty with night vision, making night driving a problem. People also complain of less tolerance to sunlight.

Many people I have spoken to who had refractive surgery now need reading glasses. They have found themselves swapping long distance glasses for close-up glasses. So many of us have jobs these days where reading or other close-up work is necessary. I know a man in his early 50s, a pianist, who spends his days reading music at the piano. He was excited to have the laser surgery to correct his myopia and now, while he doesn't need glasses for walking around or socializing, he has presbyopia and has to wear his glasses all day while he plays — an activity during which he previously sometimes left his glasses off altogether. Although he felt as though he was 'trading up', this doesn't seem to me like an improvement — at least not in a fundamental sense.

After these operations the eye remains myopic, that is, elongated towards the back and contracted towards the front. The visual cortex is still contracted, with resulting contraction in the rest of the visual system. All that has happened is that instead of glasses on the outside to compensate for the shape of the eye, the cornea has been permanently altered, thus fixing for life an area that may hinder the movement in the frontal area of the eyes. This frequently leads to presbyopia. The conjunctiva and cornea relate to the neck, throat and shoulder area. Thus a laser eye operation can — long-term — cause physical problems in the torso, neck and head beyond those caused by the dysfunction the surgery was performed to treat. The limbic system and the corpus callosum can be adversely affected which can create different problems over time.

In the future more refractive operations will be available. In general they will allow people to see more clearly but the overall coordinating mechanism and the multiple functions of the visual system may be compromised, and this may result later on in serious dysfunctions in brain, eye and body. No re-education of the visual system and its multiple functions has taken place and the original cause is still 'alive', only more subdued or hidden. We start to lack the sensitivity to notice things deteriorating.

Personally I would opt for an operation only if it were really necessary, such as after an accident if surgery is needed to save vision. I would then work on re-educating my visual system so that the emotional trauma could be dealt with together with my underlying habits. This would ensure that the natural mechanism could function again to its maximum potential even after an operation.

If you have already had refractive eye surgery, you can still re-educate your visual system, perhaps not to see more clearly, but to increase your awareness of your visual system and to enhance your overall coordination and well-being.

Emergency operations

Accidents happen. Operations following accidents are often vital to save eyesight. In the case of detached retinas, for example, it is very important to seek medical advice immediately — a laser operation will help the choroid and the retina function together again. But then some time *after* the operation it is important to undo tensions and contractions which have resulted from the operation itself, to undo the tension which caused the retina to detach in the first place, and to re-educate the visual system to prevent recurrence.

After an accident the eyes and body will compensate for the affected area in some way, creating imbalances. In other words, secondary outcomes may develop as a result of the accident and the operation. When people start to engage in this work they consciously reconnect areas of the brain with the eyes and body. Over time this will affect the structure and function of fluids within the eye; it will improve physical alignment, general health and the functioning of the reptilian brain, limbic system and neocortex. Education also brings increased awareness into day-to-day activities like reading, walking and eating.

Case histories on visual dysfunctions

Note: Please refer to the colour foldout map inside the back cover of this book for connections relating to the Eyebody Patterns.

Myopia: Where the world is blurry in the distance

Myopia (near- or short-sightedness) originates out of a contracted upper visual cortex and is one of the most common visual dysfunctions in our modern world. Usually glasses, contact lenses or laser surgery are used to deal with myopia. Myopia tends first to appear in childhood and teenage years and its onset is seldom after age 21.

Myopia is emblematic of the contracted upper visual cortex pattern. The upper visual cortex contracts onto the limbic system which then presses against the reptilian brain. As a result of this the auxiliary areas of the eye will tighten, followed by a tightening of the frontal area of the eye. The pressure on the third ventricle causes the pupil, retina and choroids to contract. The panoramic part of the retina receives less light and the panoramic photoreceptors transmit less stimulation to the thalamus. The thalamus then deflates and moves back and down, pulling the optic nerves along with it. This creates an elongated eyeball.

Accompanying this is a shortening or tightening of the corresponding areas of the body: the lower back and the organs of digestion, followed by tension around the pelvis, the hips, the upper legs and the knees. When seated, the lower back may slump and there may be a tendency to cross the legs. In walking, the knees or legs might hurt. There may be digestive or reproductive problems. Emotionally the pattern might be experienced as anxiety, fear or feeling unsafe. The degree of such emotions will vary and may reflect the degree of myopia.

Generally speaking the spinal column will be somewhat shortened in the area of the pelvis and lower back, affecting the nerve connections to the surrounding organs and legs — this may also affect circulation in the legs. All in all, the pattern of myopia is found within the back part of the eye and the visual pathways within the brain, and the lower area of the torso and the legs, all the way to the feet.

To reverse this condition we need to build up the connection to the reptilian brain through panoramic awareness of the retina, the layer of the choroid all the way to the lens, the vitreous humour and the pathways to the reptilian brain, before we can establish the connection to the limbic system (frontal area of eyes) and the upper visual cortex (auxiliary area of the eyes). With conscious depth perception we can integrate the visual system, including the fovea centralis and the lower visual cortex for focused sight.

Case history: Myopia

Katrin was short-sighted, and in her early 30s. She told me on the phone that she had been wearing glasses since age 12. She was fed up with wearing them and had considered laser surgery but intuitively rejected it. She had heard from a friend that I helped people to re-learn how to see without visual aids. This intrigued her enough to make an appointment.

As Katrin sat in the chair opposite me the first thing I noticed was her rather stooped posture, crossed and generally heavy legs and upper torso. Her glasses were weighing her down. She gave me her eyeglass prescription — 3.75 dioptres in her left eye and — 3.50 dioptres in her right eye. Additionally the left eye had astigmatism of — 1.25 dioptres.

Katrin told me that she first saw fuzzily in school and had trouble reading the blackboard. At the same time she complained of headaches and a stiff lower back. A teacher commented that Katrin's eyes seemed strained and suggested she have them tested. Her mother took her to an optometrist, who diagnosed slight myopia. He prescribed glasses and although she didn't like wearing them in the beginning as she felt they made her somewhat lazy in her brain and eyes, she got used to them and soon wore them every day. Her headaches got better, but her lower back continued to bother her. It didn't take long before she needed stronger glasses.

Katrin couldn't remember when the astigmatism first appeared. It might have come gradually, she said. During her senior school years she was very conscious of glasses and hated wearing them, especially when dating. Later she got contact lenses, but after a few years was unable to wear these as her eyes got sore and she reverted to glasses.

Now married, Katrin told me that after the birth of her second child she was very tired and her eyes deteriorated. But after a few months she was able to see through her glasses again as well as before.

I asked her about her body. She told me her lower back always bothered her. She had occasional treatments of chiropractic, osteopathy or physiotherapy which relieved the pain. But the problem was still there, and resurfaced when she was tired or stressed. Lately her upper back had been giving her problems, and she noticed her breathing was shallower. She complained her legs were heavy. A keen runner, she had injured both knees. Otherwise she felt healthy and well.

Asked about any differences between the left and right sides of her body, she said she noticed her left side was always stiffer than the right and her left shoulder somewhat bothered her. But over the years she had ignored the little aches and pains and just kept on going.

In addition to raising her children Katrin worked in human resources for a large corporation. Her time at work was split between administration using computers and talking on the phone, lecturing to groups and consulting with people.

She said she sometimes got stressed, frustrated, and angry and felt she was on an emotional rollercoaster. She often felt overwhelmed trying to juggle her family commitments, work and personal interests. She felt supported by her husband, although their lives had drifted a little apart. She was not overly concerned about this, although it was at the back of her mind.

Anxiety had always been part of her life. Not that she noticed it every day, but she recalled times before school tests or meeting people when there was a sense of worry and nervousness about performing well and not failing. She tried hard to achieve in all areas of her life.

During our first sessions we worked on establishing a sense of her retina and vitreous humour, which helped greatly to ease her lower back discomfort and also increased her sense of security.

She realized that she didn't need to wear glasses from morning till night, and started leaving them off at home. She commented that she was seeing fuzzily but that after a few days she felt fine about it — she didn't have to see everything totally clearly. Her impression was that she was able to see enough to do what was needed: prepare dinner, watch TV (sitting more closely than before), listen to music and plant flowers in the garden.

We continued the lessons by establishing a relationship with Katrin's optic nerve, the highway from the eye to the brain. She got the sense of making contact with the optic nerve, and the brainstem moving more freely forwards and up.

She noticed her running improving: "I was running my normal stretch of kilometres and the last two times I was not even panting, I could have run far longer. While I was running I thought about my optic nerves connecting more upwards around my brainstem and somehow my legs felt much lighter and easier. My head was lighter, my vision was clearer — but the best thing was I didn't feel exhausted afterwards."

We were ready for the next step. I guided her from the eye, via the rising optic nerves, connecting to the back area of the brainstem, then through the thalamus and limbic system to the upper visual cortex. From the upper visual cortex at the back of the skull Katrin then visualized the entire visual pathway for integrating the whole system. We worked on conscious depth perception; this took a bit of practice and each session Katrin left with some homework, like making dinner or looking at her computer screen with conscious depth perception. Katrin quickly realized that she could apply conscious depth perception in many areas and she noticed the changes.

She became aware of a new way to deliver her presentations and said she felt much more 'in tune' and present, more able to 'hold' her audience. In a similar way she felt that her connection with her husband changed in quality and he noticed that she seemed more available in their relationship. To her astonishment not only did her running become faster, but she started to notice many more shapes and colours while running, seeing her surroundings with more and more clarity.

Katrin came less frequently as she became more familiar with the principles of the vision work and could apply techniques in her daily activities to see better and release tensions within her visual system and body. She no longer wears glasses.

Presbyopia: Where the arms are too short to read the newspaper

Blurry eyesight is usually first noticed reading in dim light. This gradually worsens and straining to see and over-focusing becomes the norm.

Presbyopia, or middle-age vision, occurs from around age 40. It is conventionally believed that the ability of the lens to accommodate by means of its surrounding ciliary muscles is lost, so close-up vision blurs. My own understanding is that the loss of ability to accommodate is due to the deterioration of primary functions within the visual system with specifically a narrowing or overextending of the frontal area of the eye (depending on the upper visual cortex type). The lens continues to grow throughout our lives and there is ongoing intrinsic movement within the lens and lens fluid — losing this mobility is not an inevitable part of the ageing process as is commonly thought.

Presbyopia can occur in both the contracted and the overextended upper visual cortex types. In the case of the contracted type, the front area of the eye will tighten, leaving the lens and its fluid compressed. In the case of over-extension, the frontal area and lens over-widens, straining the front by pulling it tight. By neglecting the overall coordination of the visual pathway, individual areas within the eye malfunction; some work harder, some less, and over time the system becomes fatigued.

The usual pattern is that we finally give in, go to an eye specialist to get glasses, or try a pair of supermarket glasses that give us clear sight close-up. The consequences, although subtle and often not noticed, are that our brain gets used to the glasses and the need to wear them becomes stronger. The dependency flourishes and the whole brain becomes less involved in the process of seeing.

My experience is that the lens has a correlation with the diaphragm. When the structures surrounding the lens (the vitreous humour, ciliary process and its attached small muscles, the aqueous humour fluid and the cornea) are not moving freely, the lens has difficulty maintaining its subtle movement and the fluid within it stagnates. When presbyopia occurs there are likely to be breathing difficulties and the body will show signs either of slumping in the upper back with a collapsing chest (contracted upper visual cortex type), or a rigid way of holding the chest area tight and sometimes overly upright (overextended type).

Looking at the larger picture, presbyopia has much to do with the ability to make contact with the outer world. The loss of lens function can create a sort of barrier between our inner and outer environment. It may give us the opportunity to rethink our vision from age 40.

Case history: Presbyopia

James attended one of my six-day retreats. On the introductory evening he shared his story of his arms becoming too short to read the newspaper. We all cracked up because he spoke with such humour and many in the circle nodded their heads in empathy. He described how so many of his friends took their glasses out as soon as the restaurant menu was placed upon the table, or when they needed to look up numbers in the telephone book. The 6's, 8's and 9's were jumbled up and his brain no longer had any idea what to make of them. When I asked him about his body and physical habits he mentioned that his wife pulled him up sometimes as she noticed he slumped in his chest much more than he used to. Now in his mid-40s, he felt generally healthy and normal though his breathing seemed to have deteriorated in recent years. He was aware of being much more out of breath working out at the gym. But only the glasses really bothered him.

After about a year of trying to avoid glasses he finally gave in and now had numerous pairs strategically placed so that he could always find one. He had them beside each telephone in the house, on his desk close to his computer, on his car dashboard and in his office. The first two pairs he bought at a chemist, then purchased the others from the supermarket. He felt well equipped with glasses — and had a huge smile on his face when he said how ridiculous he felt to be surrounded by them and dependent on them. He was at the workshop because he was sure there must be a better and more natural way to deal with his vision problem.

It was clear to me that James had to learn first and foremost to use his upper visual cortex, which was the contracted type. He was so 'forward' in his eye that his brain did not do the appropriate work. As I guided the whole group through the fundamentals of discovering their visual systems, James noticed an increased ability to see more clearly. Colours became brighter and outlines sharper. He was gradually able to apply conscious depth perception to objects located in the distance. When we came to the front area of the eyes he noticed an intrinsic lack of freedom and responsiveness. The vitreous humour especially seemed to push against the lens and the fluid seemed almost stagnant. He sensed how he slouched so much in his body. By freeing the front of his eyes his upper chest area, neck and head were able to move more freely and he noticed how much more comfortable it was to see and to move his head, neck and shoulders at the same time.

After some time applying these new skills we set out to tackle reading. I gave everyone a reading chart with lines in various font sizes. I asked James and the others in the group which lines were easy to read without any strain. The emphasis was not on trying hard to see everything clearly, but instead on using new skills in the visual system. For James I especially emphasized panoramic vision so that his eyes (in the front and the back) could widen. After a few moments practice he was able to distinguish the 6's, 8's and 9's in small print and read three lines further than before. He mentioned later that suddenly the black letters and numbers stood out against the white background.

James' task was to gradually foster this new way of seeing. He practised a little every day and was finally able to let go of his habit of wearing glasses. He became confident of being able to see for himself. At the same time his posture (especially his lower and upper back) became increasingly more aligned and his breathing improved as the frontal tension of the eyes gradually reduced. As James said at the end of the workshop: there is no need for glasses at all, regardless of age.

James took follow-up individual lessons with me after the workshop. These have helped him deepen his experiences so that he has become more confident applying his new skills. He also purchased a pair of pinhole glasses to use if he is extremely tired to see just a little more clearly and to exercise the panoramic function of his retina. I often recommend the use of pinhole glasses in presbyopia, especially during a transition period, to see clearly and foster panoramic vision.

The process and rate of progress is different for everyone, and so are the goals. Some people only want to reduce their habit of wearing glasses a little; others are more committed and apply the principles in day-to-day activities to achieve a greater improvement. I emphasize that anyone can do it: it just takes some guidance, a willingness to keep learning, and practice.

Hypermetropia: Where things appear bigger than life

This form of visual dysfunction usually shows up in childhood. It is far less common than myopia, affecting perhaps less than 10% of the population. Hypermetropia (long- or far-sightedness from an early age) relates to an overextended upper visual cortex type. Here the eyeball, generally speaking, is too wide. The fovea centralis is being bombarded by light and close-up vision is blurry.

The heart and lungs are often tight as the whole upper torso tends to be broad, with less space front to back. You may notice similarities between the overextended upper visual cortex type and hypermetropic character traits — but keep in mind that having an overextended upper visual cortex does not necessarily make one hypermetropic.

A disproportionate number of musicians, singers, dancers, designers, global leaders and entrepreneurs are in this category. They have many creative talents, and have found a way to cope with the disconnection in the close encounters that masks their vulnerability. Looking through the glasses of a far-sighted person, everything appears very, very large. This is also reflected in 'huge' internal pictures.

In hypermetropia the visual cortex is overextended and wide. This produces an over-widening of the eyeball itself, especially the closer we come to the front of the eye. The further forward we get in the visual system, the wider everything becomes. The front of the eye is associated with the external environment. The vitreous humour presses more on the lens, creating inner pressure. From a physical perspective, the liver and pancreas are affected, which can bring frustration and anger.

Generally speaking people with hypermetropia need to connect, to think 'smaller' within themselves so they can 'fit' into their own visual pathways and their own brains. I have found extraordinary changes possible by guiding hypermetropic people through this process. An inside connection occurs which seems to allow their brain to find a size which actually 'fits into the skull'. A sense of connection, peace and ease occurs, allowing them to live more easily in their eyes and body. As the overly wide limbic system finds its own integration and connection the sense of letting things come close feels far less threatening. The vision work can help soften the front of the eye, allowing clearer perception of close objects, as well as more comfort and ease in relationships.

Case history: Hypermetropia

Eileen, a tall, blonde designer in her 60s, attended one of my seminars. Seated in the back row, she explained in the introductory session that she wore glasses from age three, then took them off at puberty and never used them again. She was articulate and highly confident and said that she had always had a fascination with vision and colour. She was attending the seminar with her partner and they were both interested to learn what they could do for themselves.

After only a day she commented that she realized she had always been able to see clearly but her brain had never really taken this information in fully. "I think that is why I am really here, to learn to see from my brain so my eyes can be relaxed rather than tired and strained, especially when I do loads of close-up design work."

She was sometimes rather blunt with her partner and short-tempered. Eileen spoke about her frustration whenever things got too close: "I know I am sometimes too forthright, and this puts people off. But I don't mean to." Then Eileen mentioned that she felt as if she needed protection because everything she saw was always very big — and therefore overwhelming. "Especially when someone stands close to me, I see him or her as very big. Then I feel overwhelmed and I lash out. I was still very young when I noticed it felt so much more comfortable when people were not close to me. I guess I still keep my distance so I feel safe, and people don't dare get too close to me either." Her partner said that it didn't feel good to him, as he was the one she was often sharp with. She realized that perhaps in some circumstances this way of protecting herself might be appropriate, but not always; and not in situations where she actually wanted more intimacy.

We started working to bring the overextension more into alignment within the upper visual cortex. This allowed her gradually to experience her environment as smaller and more manageable. After a while everyone commented how much easier it was to be in Eileen's space and she herself felt much better. Her frustration lessened, her patience improved and she enjoyed closer encounters. Her partner was thrilled. From this six-day workshop they took away tools which helped them both — emotionally, physically and mentally.

Astigmatism: Have we really got two moons?

Astigmatism is caused by irregular curvatures of the cornea. The three layers of the cornea, instead of overlapping equally, become distorted. Things can appear to be doubled; in the sky there can almost appear to be two moons.

Astigmatism can be present in either upper visual cortex type. The cornea relates directly to the corpus callosum; astigmatism from a contracted upper visual cortex means the corpus callosum becomes depressed in a concave manner, while the overextended upper visual cortex pattern means the corpus callosum is being overstretched into a convex pattern. The cornea changes shape in the opposite direction of the corpus callosum in both cases.

The corresponding area in the body for the cornea is the shoulder girdle. For contracted types there may be shoulder pain or a general narrowing of the upper back. In overextended types an over-widening of the shoulder may lead to pain or discomfort and tightening in the neck and throat.

After applying the primary coordinating mechanism the frontal and auxiliary areas of the eyes need inclusion so the corneas are supported by surrounding fluids and structures and the curvature can change its shape through appropriate connections to the brain.

Case history: Astigmatism

Twenty-five year-old Samantha attended a number of my workshops. She was highly skilled and intelligent. She had slight myopia but her primary vision difficulty was astigmatism in both eyes of about —3. I immediately noticed her sense of self-protection when she first spoke up in the group.

During the following days she shared how she felt vulnerable in the presence of other people. She felt that she used her glasses as a protective mechanism to keep people out. We worked to connect with the vitreous humour to create inner safety as well as allowing the eyeball to expand from within. She quickly realized that her astigmatism was functioning as a 'protective shield' around her. She also noticed that her upper torso was very shallow and that her shoulder blades stuck out. She became aware that her shoulder blades were not really being supported by the torso underneath. Her shoulders were tight and she complained of frequent neck and shoulder tension. She had had regular chiropractic treatments which helped for a while, but her shoulders were always somewhat sore and stiff.

With a new ability to delicately allow the vitreous humour to find new places inside the eyeball, and working through the optic nerves, she experienced a greater sense of stability from the back of her visual system. Visualising the upper visual cortex and allowing the seeing process to begin from there, we worked our way gradually forward to keep a sense of expansion all the way through. This then affected the frontal fluid — the aqueous humour — which started to support the layers of the cornea.

Later on during private lessons we were able to allow more aqueous humour fluid to reach through the pupil so that the whole front area of the eye, and especially the cornea, was being supported again. The main difference she noticed was her posture, and the easing of soreness in her shoulders. Her whole upper torso gradually 'filled up' and began supporting the easing shoulders. Samantha also felt her immune system was stronger and noticed fewer infections during the winter months. On another level her sense of inner safety and being able to allow people to get closer without losing her own sense of safety became stronger. She didn't need to protect herself so much and could allow a healthier space and natural boundary between herself and her surroundings. Her astigmatism at first fluctuated and then gradually reduced to the point where she didn't need glasses any more: she no longer had the 'double moon' experience.

Glaucoma: Pressures in life

Glaucoma happens when the balance between production and elimination of the aqueous humour is out of balance. This creates pressure in the eyeball which results in damage to the optic nerve. There is a widening of the optic disc and a narrowing or over-tightening of the aqueous humour exit canal, the canal of Schlemm. The widened optic disc creates pressure on the choroid process, affecting the blood flow within it, with an overall tightening towards the front, especially at the ora serrata and towards the pupil. The canal of Schlemm is always affected; aqueous humour fluid is restricted at the exit through the canal and inner pressure builds up.

Depending on the upper visual cortex type (glaucoma is found within both types), this may lead to open-angle (overextended upper visual cortex) or closed-angle (contracted upper visual cortex) glaucoma.

After establishing the primary coordinating mechanism, people with glaucoma need to relate the visual pathway through the limbic system together with the frontal area of the eye, especially the canal of Schlemm, the optic nerves, optic discs, the retinas and the choroids to activate the thalamus.

Case history: Glaucoma

Patrick came to me for a second opinion on his glaucoma, which had just been diagnosed. His eye specialist suggested using drops as soon as possible to reduce the intraocular pressure. Patrick didn't like the idea of having to use drops for the rest of his life. He wanted to tackle the root cause rather than the symptoms of the problem.

As we started working it became clear that he was somewhat frustrated with his life. He worked as an accountant and had reached the top of his career ladder as a partner in an accounting firm. He was 50 and wasn't looking forward to spending the rest of his working life as an accountant. He had a passion for art, painting and sculpture — in fact he had been torn between studying art or accounting, and opted for the financial security of an accounting career. As we worked together over the following months he became more and more sceptical about staying in accounting.

I shared with him my experience that with glaucoma there is often an inner urge to do or be something very different in life. Hence a certain pressure builds up in the front area of the eye, reflected in our relationship to the outside world.

Patrick's physicality was typical for glaucoma and an overextended upper visual cortex. His heart and chest area were very tight. This reflects the closing of the canal of Schlemm, which inhibits the free movement of the aqueous humour and results in a build-up of fluid, creating excessive pressure.

Patrick was a very committed person. Whatever he did, he committed himself fully and did it very well. Much of his identity was invested in his profession. I supported him through a two year process until he eventually made the decision to leave his professional partnership.

He went to an art college, working in accounting during his holidays. He felt freer, more fulfilled and glad that he had made the change, although at the time it was difficult for him. His eye pressure has been stabilizing ever since. He has regular checks from his eye specialist, but for years now his inner eye pressure has been within the normal reading without drops. His awareness of his chest area, back and legs has changed dramatically, and he stands more easily than ever.

Cataracts: Gradual blurring at any distance

Cataracts can happen at any age, but mostly occur in people over 60. Sometimes they are the after-effect of an operation or a side effect of medication. A gradual calcification of the lens fluid results in blurred vision at any distance. But the lens continues to grow throughout our lives with continual intrinsic movement within the lens and lens fluid — so it is not 'necessary' to develop a cataract, despite what some may think.

The calcified lens can be removed in a relatively quick operation, and a refractive lens inserted. In other words, the glasses that would have been worn externally are now inside the eye — with the disadvantage that there is no taking them off at night.

Lens fluid calcification relates directly to a constriction in the diencephalon which, depending on the upper visual cortex type, is either the result of deflating (contracted type) or overstretching (overextended type).

From the Eyebody perspective the lens relates to the diaphragm. The lens is also the area where the inner mechanism and the outer environment meet. Even if there is a decision to go for an operation, it is vital that the underlying habits that caused the calcification be detected and gradually worked with. A frequent problem is that as soon as the cataract is removed and clear sight is restored, the commitment to continuing to work to free the eye from within is often lost.

As with all dysfunctions, establishing the primary coordinating mechanism is the first step to undo the pattern of cataracts. The frontal area of the eyes, the retina and vitreous humour need to be stimulated so that the fluids of the lens can be supported with nutrients to undo the calcification. The reptilian brain and limbic system play a major role in this, together with the efficient functioning of the pineal and pituitary glands. Even if there has been a cataract operation, it is vital for the long-term health and optimal functioning of the eye to establish the primary coordinating mechanism and prevent recurrence.

Case history: Cataract

I worked with Jane when she was in her late 60s. She had cataracts in both eyes and had opted to have them removed. The operation was successful but left her with difficulty seeing close-up, a dramatic increase in light sensitivity and a decrease in night vision. Even months after the cataract operation she felt somewhat irritable and not quite herself. Her self-esteem and general sense of self had suffered.

I asked her about her breathing, whether she had noticed any changes since the surgery. She said that she had been asthmatic as a child but it eased in her late teens. Her breathing was always poor during sport so she abandoned sporting activities quite early on. She had noticed a decrease in breathing capacity since her cataracts, but thought it was the inevitable result of getting older.

I explained the relationship between the lenses and the diaphragm. The whole front area of her eyes was extremely tight. With an old habit of tightening the front of the eye, the fluids of the aqueous humour, the vitreous humour and the lens could not function properly. Jane learned to use her retina, choroid and vitreous humour more fully and effectively. She noticed that her whole body started to change, allowing more movement and less downward slump from the upper body to the hips. Then we worked on her optic nerves, which helped her stand more upright.

After learning to relate from her upper visual cortex we then worked our way to the front of the eye via the reptilian brain and limbic system. Gradually freeing the fluids and the structures within the front of the eye helped her to use the plastic lenses inserted during the operation in a more freeing and moveable way. After some months she was able to see much more easily both during the day and the evening. Her breathing had dramatically improved and her stance had changed from collapsed to upright.

Crossed-eyes or squints: Which eye is really looking at me?

Which eye is really looking at me? That is often the question parents will ask a child with a squint. Usually the child ends up at the eye specialist who suggests an eye patch, and if that doesn't work, an operation on the extrinsic eye muscles will be performed to 'straighten out the eye'. Crossed-eyes or squint may occur without other visual dysfunction, in which case there will be clear sight. The issue then is solely the appearance of the eyes.

Crossed-eyes occur in either upper visual cortex type but are more common in cases of overextension. Sometimes only one eye turns in or out, sometimes both, or one eye may be up and the other slightly down. A combination of all these is possible. The underlying cause appears to be a lack of fusion within the thalamus, close to the third ventricle. Especially in hypermetropia, both sides of the thalamus seem to over-widen. This causes a lack of coordination from the thalamus, forwards through the optic nerves and the optic chiasm to the eyes themselves.

The six extrinsic eye muscles connected to the outer sheath of the optic nerve tighten, causing the eye to turn.

We don't really have to change anything about the extrinsic eye muscles; instead we need to learn how to restore the upper visual cortex function which will realign and coordinate the limbic system and the thalamus, with the extrinsic eye muscles following the optic nerve movement. If one of the extrinsic eye muscles is shortened in an operation the eye will look straight ahead, but fundamentally nothing changes within the brain or the optic nerve. The operation is done for aesthetic reasons; it does not improve eyesight, nor does it deal with the cause of the squint. Patching the eye can be constructive, but the upper visual cortex must be involved for fundamental change to occur. Working with squints is relatively easy as the cause is so clearly defined.

The condition is often noticeable from birth, or from early childhood. Sometimes in adults one eye turns out slightly. This may happen to a violinist who habitually keeps one eye on the strings, the other on the music. Often I find that the upper leg turns in the same direction as the eye moves and the head turns to one side to see. Cranial osteopathy can help restore the functions of membranes, increasing the flow of spinal and brain fluids and releasing tension within the sphenoid bone. If an operation has been done to correct a squint, it is still vital to learn good habits of seeing so that coordination and integration from within can take place.

Case history: Cross-eyes

Martin was a man in his 30s. Like his siblings he was hypermetropic and had a squint. As a child he wore a patch but this did not change his eye. He was in hospital ready to be operated on to rectify the squint when the eye specialist decided against surgery at the last minute (Martin did not know why). And so the eye stayed 'out'.

When Martin attended his first retreat with me he was wearing glasses and his left eye was definitely 'out'. He felt awkward and vulnerable. When he took his glasses off he felt embarrassed: "Now everyone can see my turned-out eye." As we worked with his overextended upper visual cortex, Martin gradually gained a sense of moving the eye and optic nerve from within, something he had felt never before.

Months later I met him again and forgot he had had a squint as it was not visible. He told me he could now direct his eye through his brain and said he no longer got strange looks from people.

Light sensitivity: There is too much light!

'There is too much light,' or 'I need sunglasses or else I get headaches,' are common statements from people with over-sensitivity to light. They may wear sunglasses all the time, even indoors. Light sensitivity has much to do with the photoreceptors within the retina and the layer of the choroid functioning inadequately. This means the thalamus and the pituitary and pineal glands are not working properly either. Sunglasses only reinforce the fact that the photoreceptors (especially the rods) aren't working efficiently and also inhibit the functioning of the two glands. Squinting and narrowing of the facial muscles are common and tension in the lower or upper back, accompanied by a certain fear or uneasiness of the dark. By learning to apply panoramic vision the rod photoreceptors and blood supply to the choroid layer of the eye start to function normally again, greatly reducing light sensitivity.

After establishing the primary coordinating mechanism, the retina, the choroid and its fluid and the optic pathways to the thalamus and hypothalamus need to be stimulated, along with the pineal and pituitary glands.

Case history: Light sensitivity

Barbara, a 24 year-old, came to me for help because she was very sensitive to bright light in winter as well as summer, which made her squint. Her night vision was also not good. She wore sunglasses a lot and often forgot to take them off. Apart from this Barbara had good vision both close-up and in the distance. We started working with panoramic vision through palming the hands over her closed eyelids and sunning with closed eyelids so she could learn how to use the rod photoreceptors more effectively, thus allowing the pituitary and pineal glands to function more efficiently. With her new awareness she reduced the amount of time she wore her sunglasses and her rods and choroid started to fully function. Her night vision improved and she no longer squinted in bright light. Barbara was free of sunglasses within a few weeks.

Night vision — I can't see a damn thing!

Night vision is the domain of the panoramic rod photoreceptors and the blood flow of the choroid. For people living in cities, where lights may be on all night, the panoramic photoreceptors might not be used much at all and the stimulation needed to see well at night does not happen.

Often a person has not really tried to see in the dark; sometimes fear of the dark prevented them from noticing what they could see. Night vision is a different kind of seeing — clarity and colour exist only in day vision. We can only see shapes and outlines, coupled with distinctions of lighter and darker shapes.

Night vision is vital as it directly involves the rod photoreceptors. When night vision is poor, the pineal gland is usually not working properly. One of its functions is the regulation of sleep patterns. This then affects the pituitary gland and therefore the overall hormonal rhythm.

First it is necessary to establish the primary coordinating mechanism, then to learn how to use the retina, the choroid and the optic nerve, and link into the pineal and pituitary glands. This will help to change the under-stimulation of the panoramic photoreceptors, vital for night vision.

Case history: Night vision

Bella, in her early 30s, attended a retreat and private lessons with me. She lived in London where it was light all night. When it was dark in her house she couldn't make out a single thing, so she tended to turn all the lights on. She even slept with lights on. Apart from her lack of night vision she was very light sensitive during the day. Her lower back and pelvis were slightly out of alignment, with the pelvis tilting a little forward. She mentioned that she needed only a few hours sleep at night and couldn't get to sleep before 1:00 or 2:00 a.m. She had been afraid of the dark since she was a child, and avoided direct sun during the day.

She was the overextended type, and we started bringing her attention to the panoramic photoreceptors and the layer of the choroid where the blood supports the retina with nutrients. Her experience changed gradually as she became more aware of using her panoramic photoreceptors, day and night. She started to feel safe in the dark, realizing she could recognise shapes and outlines. She had previously thought she should be able to see at night as well as she did during the day. Once she realized the differences, her fear started to diminish. She turned the lights out to sleep at night and her vision in the day started to improve. After a few weeks I suggested she draw the curtains so that the room was fully dark while she slept. Her overall sleep pattern changed; she was able to go to sleep earlier and woke up much more refreshed. She moved on to occasionally turn the lights off completely in the evenings, to practise recognizing the outlines and shapes in her living room. It started to become fun for her. On holiday she experimented with going on night walks with someone she knew. If her old fears started to return, by consciously directing her retina she was able to see more, and so her fears diminished. Her pelvis became more aligned and her whole body functioned better as her upper visual pathway and eye function were restored.

Detached retina

A detached retina is a 'detaching' of the retina from the choroid, although usually just one small section detaches, not the entire retina. If this happens an eye specialist has to be consulted immediately; this is an emergency, as there is the possibility of losing photoreceptors. Time is of the essence. Usually laser surgery is used to treat this condition.

Detached retinas often seem to happen in conjunction with an emotional stress, like a loved one dying or a sudden relationship break-up. The vitreous humour contracts or shortens very rapidly so the retina is suddenly not supported and pulls away from the choroid. Usually people work with me in the recovery stages, or even a long time later, but not in the emergency stage. The vitreous humour work is of vital importance to re-establish a healthy rapport between the retina (even after an operation) and the choroid. I often find associated problems in the lower back, the visceral organs, abdomen, pelvis and pelvic floor.

Detachment of the retina occurs primarily in the contracted upper visual cortex type. It affects the coordinating function of the thalamus and hypothalamus and their respective glands.

Case history: Detached retina

Forty-three year-old Mike attended one of my seminars. Three years earlier he had been diagnosed with a detached retina. He was in hospital the same day and laser surgery was performed. "Suddenly I was not able to see clearly, like I was no longer able to focus. It all happened within an hour or so, and I felt disconcerted and consulted an eye specialist. He diagnosed a detached retina and referred me directly to hospital for an operation. The recovery only took a few days, but I felt very vulnerable, very unlike me." Mike attended the seminar because he had noticed that his previously good vision had deteriorated markedly after the incident with his retina. After some questioning he shared that in the time just before the detached retina his life had been very stressful, with endless hours of work and very little play. He had not taken a holiday in years.

Then, out of the blue, his wife told him she had had an affair but that it had ended and she wanted to continue sharing her life with Mike. He had been so busy with his work that he had no idea. "My life was suddenly upside down, I felt betrayed and devastated." They decided to have counselling to sort out their relationship and decide how to continue. It was ten days after his wife told him about the affair that Mike had the detached retina.

Shortly after the operation he complained about severe lower back pain which he then started to address by going to the gym and having regular chiropractic adjustments. But the pain persisted. In the following month he was able to lessen his workload, attended men's gatherings and continued with the counselling. Mike said gradually his inner life, of which he had been totally oblivious, started to improve. After a year he and his wife mutually agreed to separate.

While working with Mike it became clear to me that the vitreous humour was still not supporting the retina, which affected the health of the choroid and its fluids as well as the optic nerves to the reptilian brain. This affected the overall coordination of the thalamus and tightened the limbic system. After a few days practising he noticed an increase in visual clarity and his back seemed more aligned. He said on completing the workshop that he had gained valuable tools in recognizing he could direct the movement of the vitreous humour, retina and choroid and as a result he was absolutely pain-free in his lower back. He left thrilled with the improvement in his eyesight and posture and confident he would not have another detached retina.

Dry eyes

Dry eyes are a result of over-tightening the eyelids. When the tear-producing glands are not functioning properly the tear ducts cannot work adequately. The eyelids relate to the bone structure of the skull and the lower tear ducts to the throat region, while the conjunctiva relates to the neck and the tear fluid to the vocal mechanism. Over-tightening the eyelids also influences the cornea and therefore the shoulder girdle as well. Often yawning is helpful to stimulate tear fluid (drops are not needed for lubrication), but in the long-term learning to free this frontal area of the visual system is vital for proper tear duct functioning. Dry eyes occur in both contracted and overextended upper visual cortex types.

After establishing the primary coordinating mechanism in relationship to the frontal area of the eye (especially the eyelids, conjunctivas and corneas) there can be more space and therefore less pressure against the eye. Then the fluids within the tear glands can be produced and flow consistently.

Case history: Dry eyes

Rebecca, a 40 year-old teacher, came to me for some sessions. One of her complaints was that she had dry eyes. Apart from this Rebecca had recently developed presbyopia. Her neck was very stiff and she had had asthma since childhood. She had frequent headaches. I noticed that Rebecca's head was pushed forwards, tightening her neck and shoulders. Her whole upper back area was curved forwards and her breathing was restricted.

Over the following weeks she learnt to use conscious depth perception from the upper visual cortex and was gradually able to free the frontal area of her eyes. This correlated with her awareness that her shoulders had much more space between them, her breathing was considerably improved and the range of motion in her neck increased. We worked on how to relate this to her reading and computer work. After a few sessions when I asked how her dry eyes were, she said she had not been using eye drops; in fact she had forgotten about them.

Floaters: What are those hairs doing in my eyes?

Floaters are very common. They are either debris from the retina or solid bits of vitreous humour fluid which look like small hairs. We see them as they pass in front of the fovea centralis. As the vitreous humour fluid is very subtle and responsive to our thinking process, its consistency, and therefore the floaters, can change from moment to moment. In times of emotional stress we might see more floaters and with a high degree of myopia floaters are more likely.

Tension held within the lower back is very common and the liver, kidneys, pancreas, organs of digestion and reproduction may be affected. Floaters can occur in both the contracted and overextended types.

The primary coordinating mechanism, including the limbic system and the reptilian brain, needs to work more efficiently. The vitreous humour responds by changing consistency to appropriately support the retina. This will lead to the floaters dissolving into the vitreous humour fluid and disappearing.

Case history: Floaters

Anita, in her mid-50s with strong myopia, came for sessions. She felt exhausted and heavy in herself. Her posture was short and slumped. Emotionally she was uptight. Anita noticed her floaters only when she first took off her glasses. Her vitreous humour was very tight as is the case with strong myopia. By learning to bring awareness into the visual system, and especially the vitreous humour, she gradually started to learn how to allow it to move to support her retina and the choroid. After a few sessions Anita commented that she no longer noticed so many floaters. Over time the floaters disappeared as she was more able to integrate the use of the visual system and allow her vitreous humour to move freely.

*

By learning consciously to use our visual system fully we activate our inner resources to improve overall coordination and body function. But just having inner resources is not enough to cope in a challenging world and changing environment. We need to apply them to different areas of our lives. The next chapter gives examples of how we can do this.

6

The eye to body relationship

This chapter addresses the relationships between physical dysfunction — such as back pain, heart trouble, or an old injury — and the eyes and the brain. We can discover what is happening in the visual system by looking at what's happening in the body. Please refer to the colour foldout map at the back of this book for connections relating to the Eyebody Patterns.

The eye to body relationship

We have been looking at the relationship between brain, eyes and body. There is a hierarchy in our organization: the overall coordination of the brain is at the top and the body is at the bottom. The body is made of dense matter while the brain and visual system is made of delicate tissue — think how intricate brain surgery is compared to surgery on other parts of the body. The system of organization goes from more subtle to less, so there is only a marginal improvement in the visual system or brain if we improve the body. Working through the body is not a reliable way to improve vision. Nutrition, exercise, or bodywork may improve eyesight for a while, but will not address the hierarchy from brain to eye to body. Change will only be transient when we use mechanical and external means to improve our eyesight.

Consciously working with the visual system, however, can bring lasting improvements in other parts of the body. It is a reliable way to deal with a range of postural problems and dysfunctions. The Eyebody Patterns can be used as a diagnostic tool. Concrete difficulties like lower back pain as well as less tangible things like auto-immune or hearing difficulties can be understood and changed by working through the visual system.

Frequently I work with people with clear sight. That is, I help them undo tension held in their bodies by working through the visual system; both the body and the visual system release.

Hearing and the visual system

In all of my workshops there are participants who suffer from a degree of hearing loss or the discomfort of tinnitus.

When we disconnect from our visual system to listen to the sound of speech, music or noise, we abandon the coordination of the thalamus and the connection from the optic nerve to the thalamus. Our hearing connects into the brain just beneath the connection of the optic nerves with the thalamus. By learning primarily to connect with the visual system and secondarily with our hearing, the brain can work more effectively and it becomes effortless to see and hear at the same time.

In the case of the overextended upper visual cortex the entire upper visual pathway is over-widened, leaving the audio connections over-exposed. In my experience these people usually have a love of music and are often singers, musicians or dancers. Their overextended upper visual cortex characteristics predispose them to this, but there is a danger: they tend to become overly fatigued. They can be highly sensitive to sound of any kind and often feel overwhelmed by discordant sound. The upper visual cortex (relating to the eyelids and affecting the cranial bones and the bones of the inner ear canal), the tear fluid (relating to the larynx), and the limbic system (relating to the iris and aqueous humour) are crucial links. What is needed is to guide the coordination of the visual system together with conscious depth perception to allow the cranial bone structure to integrate, especially the inner ear canal. Hearing then happens effortlessly — and three-dimensionally. If a person concentrates only on his or her hearing, the primary coordinating system is not being used and the overextended upper visual cortex continues in its pattern.

I once developed some tinnitus while flying across the U.S. on a night flight. My ear was leaning against the window and there was a constant roaring sound for over four hours. When I reached New York I was full of tinnitus. It took me a while to figure out that I had lost contact with the visual system because I was so over-burdened with the sound of the humming. By consciously coordinating the visual system, my hearing started to change and the noise in my ears eased up.

While flying I now use earplugs or noise-cancelling headphones so that I can stay with the visual system more easily. Not being drawn into the constant humming of the plane helps me to stay in contact with the visual system; this is vital to avoid jet lag.

Emotions and the visual system

Emotions originate in the structure of the brain. The limbic brain is also known as the emotional brain, and old memories are believed to be held within the amygdala. The corresponding relationship within the eye is found in the region of the iris and the surrounding fluid of the aqueous humour (which corresponds with the physical and emotional heart). Then there are those feelings relating to the reptilian brain and its fight or flight response, those of fear and anxiety, which I relate to the vitreous humour, the fluid that supports the eyeball from within. In some people this fluid can start to solidify and have little ability to move. The vitreous humour relates to the lower back as well as visceral organs like the digestive system. When I work with someone who has almost no ability to contact their vitreous humour I may refer them for psychotherapy. I then work concurrently with the therapist as the ability to access this area within the eye increases. This will have a freeing effect on the thalamus and hypothalamus and finally the coordinating mechanism passing through the limbic system is harmonized to an extent that the 'stuckness' associated with the old collected memories leaves the system altogether.

It is important to synchronize the reptilian and limbic brains so we can live as emotionally connected human beings, attentive to our environment and knowing emotionally where we stand. Using the neocortex exclusively is not enough to become socially connected and responsible. I believe that the anti-social disconnection of younger people (as well as adults) may be rooted in the lack of coordination between the reptilian and limbic brains. Engaging in the process of integrating these systems can coordinate those brain functions so that we can experience our wholeness again and learn to connect fully with others.

Physical injury and the visual system

Let's look at an example of how an injury can affect the body and, unknowingly, the visual system: seven year-old Tom gets hit by a car. He has no obvious injuries except some anxiety and lack of appetite for a day or so. After that he appears normal. Weeks later Tom says his lower back is sore. Six months later the regular eye checks at school show that Tom has difficulty reading the chart. He also mentions that he now has to sit much closer to the blackboard to see things clearly. His parents consult an optometrist and it is confirmed that Tom is myopic. He gets a pair of prescription glasses and is advised to wear them all the time. And Tom does what he is told…

Perhaps if the effects of the accident had been dealt with Tom may not have needed glasses. Fear and anxiety show up in the lower back and abdominal region, which correlate to the vitreous humour. Although Tom appeared normal a day or so after his accident, the vitreous humour was likely to have still been contracting. It takes awareness to 'undo' this. The vitreous humour supports the retina, or in this case did not support the retina, and his lower back became sore over time. The body also showed signs of fatigue, with sensory awareness numbed after a few days. Because of this the pain disappeared and he got on with life. But the vitreous humour and the retina stayed contracted and other areas in his visual system followed. Tom belonged to the contracted upper visual cortex type and therefore effects from this seemingly small accident showed up as myopia.

In a child's life there are many small, or seemingly small, accidents. These do not all lead automatically to myopia, but a really strong impact, or compounded effects over a period of time, may. The same is true of other visual dysfunctions. Tom could have been helped at any stage in this process, without having to get glasses.

The links of body to eye

The following is a list of physical issues and their links to different areas in the visual system. This list is by no means complete but will give insight into the relationship between the body and the visual system. Most are found in both contracted and overextended upper visual cortex types.

Head, neck and spine region

Hearing is linked to the eyelids and conjunctiva, to the thalamus and functions of the pituitary gland, and to a large degree to the upper visual cortex. With integration of the visual system hearing becomes a three-dimensional experience. With dysfunction in an overextended or contracted type this may lead to tinnitus and over-sensitivity to sound and noises.

Headaches, migraines, and head injuries are linked to the eyelids, especially the lower eyelids, the conjunctiva, tear duct fluid, the retina, the optic nerve (including the disc and chiasm), the thalamus, limbic system and the upper visual cortex. With integration of the visual system, the cranial structure, the fluids and the membranes of the brain are balanced and responsive.

Throat disorders, neck tension, speech impairment are linked to the eyelids, conjunctiva, cornea, aqueous humour, choroid body (with its respective connections to the thalamus and hypothalamus and the pineal and pituitary glands). A major role is played by the limbic system (especially the corpus callosum) and the upper visual cortex, with corresponding visual impairments of astigmatism, myopia, hypermetropia, presbyopia, glaucoma and cataracts. When the visual system is coordinated speech will be freer, neck and throat areas more released and balanced.

Teeth, upper and lower jaw are linked to the eyelids, especially the lower eyelids, eyelashes, conjunctiva and cornea.

The spine and spinal cord relate to the hyaloid canal. The hyaloid canal plays an important role in the embryology of the eye as it formed the lens. The function of the lens, the pineal and pituitary glands as well as the third ventricle also play a role.

Upper torso, hand and arm region

The breathing mechanism, the diaphragm and the lungs link to the lens fluid, choroid body, ciliary body, retina and vitreous humour. They also directly link into the coordination of the thalamus and hypothalamus (and respective glands), along with the third ventricle and its pulsating spinal fluid, which becomes part of the limbic system. Dysfunction may lead to cataracts, presbyopia, myopia and glaucoma.

Heart and associated disorders link to the iris and its surrounding structures and fluids — the aqueous humour, lens, ciliary body, choroid, vitreous humour and retina. The iris is linked to the fornix within the limbic system. Heart problems can arise in either upper visual cortex type.

Shoulders, arms and hands: tension in the shoulders and upper back, shoulders hunched forward, pains in arms, numb hands and fingers, pins and needles in hands, poor blood circulation in hands and cold hands are linked to the frontal part of the eye, the sclera, and the outer sheath of the optic nerves. These physical dysfunctions show up in hypermetropia, myopia, presbyopia and astigmatism and are found in both upper visual cortex types.

Lower torso region

Visceral organs, organs of digestion, pancreas, liver, spleen are linked predominantly to the vitreous humour and the retina; the choroid body, the thalamus and hypothalamus and their respective glands also play a role. Difficulties in these areas can be present in myopia, presbyopia, hypermetropia and glaucoma and can occur in either upper visual cortex type.

Lower back pain, menstrual tension, and reproductive disorders are linked to the vitreous humour, retina, choroid, fovea centralis, cone and rod photoreceptors, optic chiasm, and relate to the thalamus and hypothalamus with their respective glands. These difficulties occur especially with myopia, presbyopia and glaucoma.

Hip joint region

Hip joint pain and pain in the groin area, lower back pain, and pelvic imbalances, are linked to the optic disc (the connection where retina, choroid and optic nerves meet), the retina, choroid, vitreous humour, and optic nerve and the thalamus, hypothalamus and their respective glands and the lateral geniculate bodies. This region is associated with glaucoma, myopia and hypermetropia in both upper visual cortex types.

Upper leg and knee region

Varicose veins, shortened leg, painful menstrual cycles, knees turning in, more body fat at hip level are linked to the optic nerve, retina, choroid body, pituitary and pineal glands and the thalamus and lateral geniculate bodies. This is seen especially in hypermetropia, crossed-eyes, glaucoma, presbyopia and myopia.

Lower leg and feet region

Bunions, shin disorders, feet turning in or out, high/low arches, are linked to the lower visual radiation (between the lateral geniculate bodies and the lower visual cortex) and the lower visual cortex. These difficulties are found especially in crossed-eyes, myopia, and hypermetropia and are therefore present in both upper visual cortex types.

Other conditions

The following conditions collected at workshops over the years detailing functional and behavioural dispositions can, at their core, be attributed to lack of upper visual cortex coordination.

Immune deficiency, general fatigue, exhaustion and depression are linked to the cornea, aqueous humour, canal of Schlemm, choroid, ciliary body and vitreous humour and show in the corpus callosum, limbic system and the reptilian brain with the thalamus, hypothalamus and their respective glands. There are links to myopia, hypermetropia and presbyopia.

Menopause, menstrual cycle irregularity and hormone functions are linked to the pituitary gland, choroid (less blood reaching the choroid), lack of presence in the retina. Rectifying this helps to ease tension in the lower back during menstrual cycles. The reptilian and limbic brains are also involved.

Sleep problems: waking during the night is linked to the pineal gland function and the vitreous humour. The reptilian and limbic brains are involved.

Blood circulation is linked especially to the fluids and fluid building properties through the choroid and ciliary body, and the reptilian brain.

Feeling safe and emotional boundaries are linked to the functions of the vitreous humour, the lens, the pupil and the frontal areas of the eye. The relevant primary area of the brain in these issues is the reptilian brain, but the limbic system and neocortex are also involved.

Scoliosis and spinal dysfunctions are linked to the thalamus/ hypothalamus and the pineal and pituitary glands, the hyaloid canal through the vitreous humour and the nasal side of the eyes. Relevant areas of the brain are the reptilian and limbic areas of the visual system, especially around the third ventricle.

Brain function, cell building, brain integration and memory are linked to the entire visual pathway. Conscious depth perception links the reptilian brain, limbic system and neocortex of the visual system and coordinates each area's brain function.

Dyslexia is linked especially to the optic nerves and the thalamus. Relevant areas are found within the reptilian brain and limbic system.

Speaking, voice production and singing difficulties are linked to the vitreous humour, lens, aqueous humour and the auxiliary areas of the eye (conjunctiva, eyelids, tear ducts and tear fluid). Relevant areas of the brain are the reptilian brain, limbic system and neocortex.

*

In the next chapter we will look at how the Eyebody Patterns can be applied to activities of all sorts, putting the principles to practical use.

7

Application to life

Application in day-to-day activities

We carry out many activities in a typical day: talk on the phone, take the dog for a walk, watch TV, present at business meetings, make love, drive in traffic, carry bags, meditate, work on computers, read manuscripts, play a round of golf, enjoy a candlelit dinner, ride a horse, work out at the gym, weed the garden — and smell the roses. Our daily life is full of continuous thought, movement and visual input. We hear, smell, taste and touch countless times throughout the day — even if we are not aware of it.

Sitting here, reading these lines in the book, the eyes and retina have to function, the brain has to comprehend and understand the contents, arms and hands have to hold the book. A vast amount of stimulus passes from moment to moment into our system. We are only conscious of a fraction of what happens behind the scenes. Most of it is hidden in our hard drive and software.

For instance, if you decide to go into the kitchen and cook a meal because you are hungry, you start visualizing what you will have to eat — either a whole picture or some details of ingredients may come to mind. Then your brain's decisions and intentions guide your eyes to see your way and your body follows to the kitchen. Many hundreds of other impulses, thoughts, movements and impressions are probably being digested by the whole system as you carry out this rather simple task of preparing your meal. Then the phone rings — and the constant processing continues.

With conscious depth perception I can direct, like the director of a play, this seemingly continuous processing facility. Without interfering with or shortcutting this inner ability to coordinate, I apply conscious depth perception from my upper visual cortex so that the neocortex, limbic system and reptilian brain can all work together and without interference at their individual tasks.

This means the activities I engage in become effortless. All aspects of the brain are coordinated; the body operates with less effort and the emotions are in synch with it all. My sensory awareness also increases, reflecting my availability for spiritual understanding.

When I bring the visual pathway into my awareness, then brain, eyes and body work together. I know it is not easy changing the habits of a lifetime. But learning fundamental approaches to better use of the brain, eyes and body can gradually be applied in our daily activities. It's fun to learn, too, as you can see the gradual improvements as you go. Step-by-step, without having to be perfect, you learn to monitor and adjust thinking, seeing and moving.

Communication is an enormously important application. We communicate with our partners, our children, with colleagues, friends and foes; we communicate our intentions during business meetings, on stage, as a teacher in class, personally and publicly — and mothers, fathers, siblings and teachers communicate with babies, toddlers, teenagers and one another. Communication happens verbally, mentally and emotionally, with our bodies, hands and arms, through the medium of a musical instrument, book, picture or sculpture. We communicate on the bus, in the office, at home, on the sports field. We participate in many forms of communication throughout the day and night — our visual system is constantly engaged.

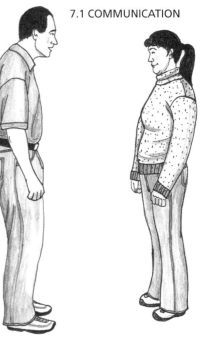

7.1 COMMUNICATION

How effective is my communication? Am I being heard? Why can I communicate with some people better than with others? How much effort do I use to communicate my intentions (and am I aware of them)?

Why is seeing so important to our communication? Because the mechanism of vision not only allows us to see clearly but also coordinates our whole self. The better we are coordinated the better we function, and the better we function the better we communicate. Our communication will only be received as effectively as it is delivered; having a well-integrated visual system ensures that we can make our intentions known clearly.

7.2 DRIVING:
contracted type

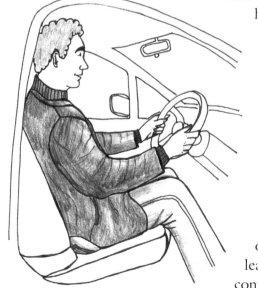

7.3 DRIVING
with panoramic vision

Let us distinguish here between the overextended and the contracted upper visual cortex types in communication (see figures 7.1). The overextended type tends to be articulate, well spoken, aloof, not miss a beat in conversation, and has a tendency to get overwhelmed and respond brashly if things get too intimate. During a conversation the mind wanders into the far corners of the universe. Others might experience the overextended character as cold, unapproachable, intolerant. Here the upper visual cortex needs to come closer together, for alignment right at the brain's coordination centre. Then with awareness applied to the brainstem, the overextended type can feel more centered: thalamus, hypothalamus, brainstem and spinal cord are aligned, and the front of the eye then aligns so that the feeling of being overwhelmed disappears — instead there is a sense of inner safety. The shoulders, neck, bone structure of the skull, and the region around the heart soften and feel relaxed. There is the feeling of a burden being taken off one's heart. Others sense an approachability, a new sense of presence, of a kind-hearted person with whom people like to communicate, who has time and knows clearly from the inside where healthy boundaries lie.

The contracted type may waffle, perhaps through anxiety or fear. A lot of effort is used to communicate ideas, striving for an outcome, and there is difficulty in making feelings clear. The nature of the contracted type is to have meagre mental images and perhaps mental chatter, without clarity of intention in communication. There is a tightening and collapsing of the brainstem and spinal cord which leads to physical slumping, drawing in, contracting the vitreous humour away from

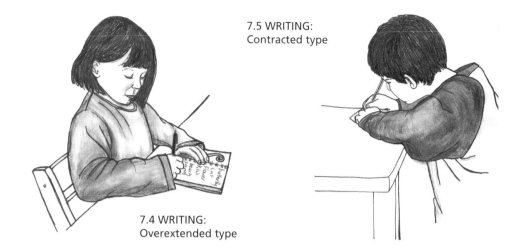

7.5 WRITING:
Contracted type

7.4 WRITING:
Overextended type

the retina, and the front of the eye collapsing. The upper body shrinks, breathing becomes shallower, the neck, throat, shoulders and head tighten. By undoing this visual pattern the whole of the visual system can open out from the vitreous humour (which relates to feelings and emotions) to the retina, to the brainstem, with the upper visual cortex expanding, so that intentions are clear and can be communicated well, with a presence and self-confidence that is clear and felt by everyone around.

Just as the overextended person can soften to come to know his/her centre from within, the contracted visual cortex person can expand in all directions without anxiety or fear, to communicate on all levels.

Applying the principles to daily activities

Here are some of the activities participants in my retreats have commented on:

Driving a car in panoramic vision keeps the driver more alive and attentive and is safer for the passengers and other drivers on the road (see figures 7.2 & 7.3).

Children at home and school may benefit enormously from panoramic vision and conscious depth perception. Many kids slouch over their desks, their schoolwork, and computer games, completely neglecting their visual system, posture, and emotional well-being. In working with children of all ages I have noticed their brain and body functions becoming more coordinated, enhancing their ability to think and see more clearly. Learning to use panoramic vision and conscious depth perception supports both creative and factual thinking, helps reduce dyslexia, encourages leaving glasses off rather than getting into a daily habit of using them, and improves general posture and body function. This work also increases the child's ability to become emotionally present and balanced and socially responsible; to be aware of themselves and attentive to their environment while feeling supported in their daily activities and developmental path in life (see figures 7.4, 7.5 & 7.6).

7.6 WRITING
with panoramic vision

Reading is a central activity in our modern world. The ability to read and assimilate information easily is an increasingly important in daily life. Many people report that reading is a leading cause of eyestrain. How we read depends largely on habits established when we first learnt how to read, as reading and language are tremendously habitual –the underlying process is unconscious. The tendency is often to over-focus on the letters, the words and the meaning alike, which results in strain and interferes with comprehension. Panoramic vision is vital for effective reading and comprehension. Applying conscious depth perception to reading allows the visual accommodation (especially the lens fluid) for near and far seeing to be fully engaged and to fully coordinate the brain. In speed reading peripheral seeing is stimulated, and this can also be applied to normal, every day reading.

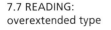

7.7 READING:
overextended type

Often during my retreats people comment on how much clearer the words seem and how their comprehension improves. Pinhole glasses can be very useful in presbyopia for improving the reading process. (see figures 7.7, 7.8 & 7.9)

7.8 READING:
contracted type

Using a computer is for many of us a daily activity – and one in which strain and frustration are often experienced. Those with myopia can enlarge fonts to decrease

94

eyestrain, but it is far more useful to learn how to use the visual system in a coordinated, efficient manner to allow overall optimal functioning of eyes, brain and body. As with reading, panoramic vision is the starting point. This coordination from the upper visual cortex integrates brain and body and therefore any eyestrain or physical fatigue (especially in the upper back, shoulders, arms, wrists, hands and lower back) can be consciously attended to and eliminated. (see figures 7.10, 7.11 & 7.12)

7.9 READING
with conscious depth perception

7.10 COMPUTING:
contracted type

As a flight passenger, pilot or flight attendant, jet lag can, to a large extent, be prevented as sleep patterns are regulated through awareness of the pineal and pituitary glands. Sleeping on a plane becomes easier for passengers.

For musicians, playing or singing by heart seems to be much easier and more coordinated than reading music; in reading music there can be a tendency to over-focus on the notes and the quality may not be as good. This is observable to the player and the audience as well. As an instrumental musician, coordinating the visual system through conscious depth perception gives the possibility of playing effortlessly whilst listening and reading music three-dimensionally. For singers, it increases the presence of the singer and their vocal resonance, and increases the ability to hear and see the music. The results are effortless breathing, coordination of the vocal mechanism and an increased ability to engage with the audience. For singers and solo or orchestral musicians with an overextended upper visual cortex, performance anxiety is greatly reduced with this increased ability to stay

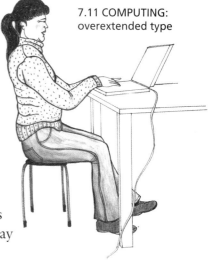

7.11 COMPUTING:
overextended type

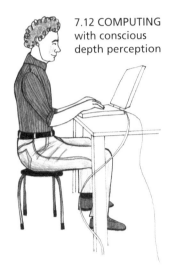

7.12 COMPUTING with conscious depth perception

centred and attentive. Subtle movement of the vitreous humour in relation to the retina, the choroid and the lens will reduce inside pressure and anxiety and help to release the holding of the breath. The use of glasses or contact lenses reduces the inclusion of the entire visual system and may restrict the overall coordination of the various areas of the brain needed for effortless performance (see figures 7.13 & 7.14).

For stage performers and professional speakers the ability to connect with the audience is vital. Conscious depth perception will increase the presence of a performer, and the listener will be able to 'come closer' to the performer. The listener will feel included in the mind and action of the performer regardless of whether five or fifty thousand people are present.

For actors and presenters in film and television the ability to use their visual system effortlessly will free the facial, neck and shoulder muscles, allowing a more natural expression of intentions or emotions. A free visual system means letting go of habitual protective armouring and enhances the ability to see and be seen naturally, while still having one's boundaries intact. Safety is of great importance and a well-functioning visual system will supply this for us naturally. Often I can detect presenters or actors who wear contact lenses or have had laser eye surgery. As the viewer, I feel excluded as they perform without the ability to be seen fully. Contact is lacking. This is very evident with camera work. The ability to use conscious depth perception will reach viewers directly and engage their interest.

For dancers the ability to move in a coordinated manner with a high degree of presence and authenticity is of the essence. Learning to use conscious depth perception from the upper visual cortex allows vision to lead the eyes and body movements intrinsically and extrinsically, thus bringing more presence and style into performances. It can also help prevent injuries. Many dancers have an overextended upper visual cortex. By connecting the upper visual cortex with the entire visual

7.13 PLAYING VIOLIN: Contracted type

system the brainstem and spinal cord align, affecting all physical movements. Injuries and excessive tensions, especially around the neck, shoulders, upper and lower back, are reduced.

Playing sports: for the professional or amateur athlete improving performance and preventing injuries are both very important. Glasses or contact lenses may hinder, or even exclude us from certain sports and may also decrease exactly what we would like to increase: stamina, speed, presence, attention to detail, efficiency of breathing, relaxation in activity, effortlessness and brain-eye-body efficiency and coordination — all important aspects of our personal performance. Skills can be honed to a much deeper level with the proper coordination of brain, eye and body.

Team sports: Playing soccer, cricket, basketball, rugby, football, water polo and other team sports provides an excellent opportunity to apply the technique of playing from the visual system individually as well as collectively. In some cases it can make the difference between winning and losing a game. By consciously using the visual system, players will increase their performance through the alignment of brain, eye and body coordination, resulting in higher speed, increased natural response mechanisms, and less injury and fatigue. If all players on a team can play from their visual system a synergy is created which is difficult to beat, awesome to watch and talked about for years to come. Trainers can experience and learn the techniques themselves along with the players. This is the best way to create team synergy, increase motivation and lead the individual players to apply the vision techniques.

Golf is a classic example of how coordination of the brain, eye, and body are vital for any swing, and for the outcome of the game. Any tension held within the visual system will tighten, collapse or over-widen the eye, the visual system and the body. Many golfers over 40 are presbyopic, and are thus misusing the lens, the lens fluid and the frontal areas of the eyes. This directly affects the upper back, neck, shoulder and breathing mechanism — and the golf swing will likewise suffer. By learning to direct through the visual system, the brainstem and spinal cord will align, improving the head, neck and back relationship, the extension of the arms, the bending of the knees (reflecting the ability to connect the optic nerves with the thalamus), as well as the ability to track the ball. The rate of accuracy increases dramatically when one learns to systematically include the visual system. Practice starts not at the driving range or at the start of a game, but while still at home reading the newspaper, including your entire visual system so not only your reading becomes easier, but also your head, neck and back coordinate. By the time you tee off you are fully present and have already coordinated your visual system. Just continue practising this and apply the visual awareness to swinging your club throughout the game. As an enthusiastic golf player once told me, finding a missing ball with panoramic vision is like seeing a white flower in the midst of a bush of red roses; the flower stands out without my trying to see it or over-focusing. The brain recognizes it and the eyes and body follow the brain's intention (see figures 7.15 & 7.16).

7.15 PLAYING GOLF: Contracted type

Working out at a gym: Many of us exercise to be fit, lose weight or just to feel better. Pumping iron, treadmilling and sweating might be a great pastime, but I don't know that they really undo inner tensions or change habits of tightening and contracting. Frequently I work with people to apply conscious depth perception while they are on the treadmill or the rowing machine, boxing or lifting weights. They notice that not only does the visual system start to function, but also their presence and performance levels increase. They can lift heavier weights, run or row faster, for longer. Watching television or reading the newspaper on the bike (because you are bored) in focused vision may rapidly decrease your ability to perform well during your workouts. Applying panoramic vision will enhance your performance and increase your attention to what you are doing — and out goes the boredom.

Walking and running are great activities. When time permits I test myself to see if I am still able to run a few kilometres, which I did regularly some years ago. I call it 'running from the visual system': I apply conscious depth perception in motion, using panoramic vision within the retina. This enables the pelvis and legs to be aligned through the central visual system and also the upper torso, neck and head to be balanced through the subtlety of the brainstem and spinal cord alignment. For me running is a great way to apply the visual system in motion, exercising mind and body simultaneously. Glasses or contact lenses leave aside panoramic vision, which leads to tension in the lower back and hip joint area as well hindering the intake of oxygen. The active visualizing capacity found within the upper visual cortex and conscious depth perception applied to the visual system sets a synergistic relationship in motion which is as effortless as being in the zone — and vital if you want to be the first past the finishing line (see figures 7.17, 7.18, 7.19 & 7.20).

7.16 PLAYING GOLF with conscious depth perception

Tennis and squash: For the racket player the ability to move quickly, to respond instantly to slight variations in the opposing player's game, stamina, and strength are all crucial for a successful game. Brain-eye-hand-body coordination is the key to tennis and squash. The ability to follow the game panoramically with minimum attention to the ball allows the rod photoreceptors to function, so the whole body can follow without our having to think where the hands and body are. Visual coordination allows arms, torso, body and legs to be in the right place at the right time. Players' comments have been "I feel relaxed and yet fully attentive, I feel in control of the game." Lower back, neck and shoulder pains, and tennis elbow can be present in both upper visual cortex types. Wearing glasses or contacts may slow responsiveness and increase the likelihood of injuries because the visual pathway is not included and there is a disconnection from the body, especially in the hip/groin area, lower back, upper legs and knees. This then prevents the upper torso from being aligned and requires more effort on the player's part, especially in the arm and upper body musculature.

Martial arts: Tai chi, karate, taekwon-do and many other martial arts are excellent activities in which to practise these principles. Because of the awareness demanded and the direction of mental and physical energy, the visual system can easily be incorporated. Unfortunately some martial arts practitioners wear glasses or contact lenses; these act as lids to the

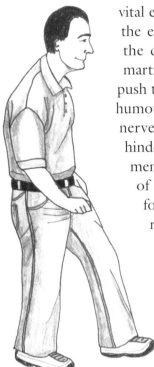

vital energies radiating through the visual system and into the environment. Glasses or contact lenses detract from the dynamic balance, strength and spiritual awareness martial artists may be seeking. In tai chi beginners often push their pelvis forwards, which is a result of the vitreous humour, retina, choroid and the connection of the optic nerves being misaligned within the visual system. This hinders the balanced coordination of emotional, physical, mental and spiritual energies. I recommend the inclusion of panoramic vision and attentiveness (versus over-focusing), allowing the pelvis to move more freely in relationship to the hip joint and the upper legs. Observing martial arts masters, I am in awe. They embody for me a beautiful dynamic sense of visual awareness, absorbed during a lifetime of practice in their discipline.

7.17 WALKING:
Contracted type

Yoga: Yoga is about 'uniting' on all levels, and including the visual pathway is an excellent way to deepen the practice. On a physical level, freeing the visual pathway creates more coordination and suppleness in the body, which allows greater symmetry and strength in any asana (pose). Freeing the lower visual cortex (overextended types) and panoramic vision within the retina (contracted types) in particular can instantly give effortless balance in one-legged poses. Leading with the visual system rather than the body supports the process of surrendering to both the sensory pleasure and the physical discomfort of yoga. The neocortex is the source of the self-doubt and mental chatter that can interfere with or subvert yoga practice, and when the balance of the reptilian and limbic brains is harmonious the mind can be quiet. This work is especially complementary to pratyahara, the drawing in of the senses. A more objective view of the inner and outer worlds is possible from the upper visual cortex. The

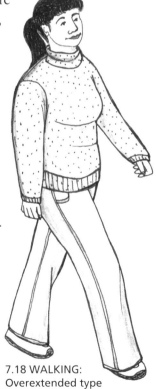

7.18 WALKING:
Overextended type

internal seat of samadhi, the ultimate stage of yoga, may well be the upper visual cortex and learning to activate it puts us readily in contact with that super-conscious state (see figures 7.21 & 7.22).

Sex and love: People with contracted visual cortexes (with their respective retinas and choroids narrower and tighter) may engage more in the outcome of sex rather than the path to lovemaking. The visual pathways give huge potential energy to the entire system and being disconnected from them leads to having sex rather than lovemaking. Learning to co-ordinate the visual system can be part of lovemaking when chosen. When the upper visual cortex is well connected and the visual system coordinated, sex and love can be simultaneously present and harmonious. This is especially important if one partner comes from the overextended camp and the other from the contracted camp. This also ties in with the emotional aspects of love.

7.19 RUNNING: Contracted type

Losing weight and eating well

When people are overweight they are often obsessed with it. There are all those thoughts about what to eat and what not to eat. By engaging with the visual system we are able to change our visual body image; the body becomes lighter as it is suspended from the visual system and the brainstem is free to move up, with the spinal cord lengthening and widening naturally. As the thalamus and hypothalamus function more effectively the associated pituitary and pineal glands work more efficiently, thus coordinating feelings of hunger, body weight, digestion and the lymphatic system. The limbic system helps on an emotional level and a sense of being nourished increases. It is then easier to choose what, when, and how much to eat. The ability to listen to the body develops around what is good for it and what to avoid, without having to continuously think about it.

7.20 RUNNING with conscious depth perception

Two types of blindness

Back in 1992 I was leading a workshop for a small group of participants. A woman, rather slumped and hunched with dark sunglasses and a white cane, was guided into the room by her son. The son left and the woman stayed for the two-day workshop. Over the two days the woman was able to recognize more and more images. With my help she began to be more upright and looked both younger and taller. She was obviously enjoying herself much more. At the end of the second day everyone in the group took a partner blindfolded through the adjoining garden for a walk as an exercise. We had not previously been in this garden, but when it was the blind woman's turn she took her partner for a walk, as everyone else had done. We were all amazed at the woman's ability to manage the walk so easily and at her uprightness and poise. When I congratulated her on her ability to do this, she didn't respond.

After completing the workshop that afternoon, the son came back to pick her up. The woman took her sunglasses out of her bag, took the cane her son gave her and slumped down as she left the venue. I have neither seen nor heard of her since.

From that day on I promised myself that I would only work with people who had the commitment to make constructive changes in their lives. I dearly hope what this woman learnt and recognized during the time we spent together helped her in some way.

Here is a totally different story. A young architect came into my office with a patch over one eye. I thought he had come to do some vision work with me, but no, he had come for some Alexander Technique lessons hoping I could help him with a sore neck. After a number of lessons I took courage to ask him what had happened to his eye. He told me that he had had a diving accident and lost his eye a few months ago. He seemed to be emotionally okay with this and able to talk about it easily. I asked if we could do some vision work. Could he include his visual pathway in his

7.21 YOGA PRACTICE
with conscious depth perception

awareness as if his missing eye was still there? With this his posture immediately changed. His neck muscles and head movement especially responded instantly. After a few more lessons with me he was excited, saying he played golf before his accident and would like to pick it up again but could not fuse his vision to track the ball. Could I help him? I suggested that he could use both his visual pathways as well as his visual cortex and gradually he was able to play golf again. Years later I met him again and he thanked me. He was still playing golf and very much enjoyed it.

It is likely that this man was using his visual system quite well before his accident and how to use it was still in his memory. If he had waited much longer his new habit of disconnecting

7.22 YOGA: contracted type

on the side on which he lost his eye would have been much stronger and perhaps no memory of the old pattern would have remained. Because he was emotionally at peace with his accident, he simply needed to see what was called for and use his consciousness and understanding to change the newly adopted habits to improve the condition quickly. He demonstrated the ability to think for himself and to implement these changes in his daily life. Of course, his eye didn't miraculously regenerate, but he could now use what he did have optimally, and that is the important thing to me — to use what I have to the best of my ability and to my full potential.

Dreams

After a retreat in Japan, a woman told me that her dreams at night were much more vivid and colourful and she could remember them with great clarity.

This often happens. When we learn to undo tension in the visual system and to direct from the upper visual cortex, a similar process of seeing continues at night. Undoing tension within the visual pathways and visual cortex as well as freeing our eyes of tension means the nightly rewiring of the brain can function more efficiently. Let me explain what I mean by the nightly rewiring of the brain. Imagine a computer: all sorts of wiring is activated inside when I turn on my laptop. I have no idea what happens as I am only an end user, not a technician. All I know is that after a grunting minute or so suddenly the screen appears and I can start work. A similar thing happens in our brain at night. Every night when we go through different sleep phases our brain is rewiring. That's why it's important that we sleep, and for enough hours, because during sleep our entire brain hardware connects anew. If we work on our visual pathways during the day, using conscious depth perception, the nightly rewiring will be different. The new pathways will help the rewiring at night and vice versa. Students of this work report that working with the visual system means sleep is much deeper and the body is lighter both at night and on waking in the morning.

Other issues

Here are some frequent issues which arise for students of the Eyebody Method:

Is exercising extrinsic eye muscles necessary?

Exercising extrinsic eye muscles is only partially helpful. What we said about the elongated eyeball in myopia, or the stiffening of the frontal area of the eyeball in presbyopia (and a combination of contractions when people wear bifocal glasses for myopia and presbyopia) means that exercising the six extrinsic muscles around the eye will make only a little difference. Unless I learn how to undo and widen the intrinsic areas of the eye and visual system, the extrinsic eye muscles will not fundamentally change. The extrinsic eye muscles are strong and have their roots in the outer sheath of the optic nerve, close to the sphenoid bone (see figure 2.5). If we learn to release the intrinsic areas of the eye, not only will the eyeball change shape from inside, but this will automatically also change the movements of the extrinsic eye muscles. Extrinsic eye muscle activities are perhaps only helpful at the start of the visual improvement process, as an extra sideline to discover the intrinsic workings of the eye. They can't do any harm but in my experience won't give the outcome some people hope for. Re-establishing clear sight requires intrinsic change.

'Being too focused '

For some participants, their interest quickens when I mention that inner vision, the spiritual aspect of developing the finer layers of the visual pathway, can be developed. I am aware that people come to this work from different perspectives, levels of engagement and personal interest.

Some come for the purely physical reason of seeing better, some to improve their posture, and some have an emotional agenda. Others are interested in developing a mental clarity or improving their brain function. Finally there are others who would like to develop the spiritual, intuitive side of seeing and an inner vision, as well as developing spiritual guidance. This is possible by applying these principles in your life.

It is vital to include the entire physical visual pathway as this will enable us to stay healthily grounded, rather than over-focusing in the body. The emotional, physical and mental aspects of the visual pathway have to be mastered first before the process of finer seeing can begin. It is vital always to come back to the physical pathway as this is the only way to not be identified with the body but still be grounded in it at the same time.

Many years ago I worked with a number of people with great clairvoyant abilities who all had long-standing myopia or presbyopia. Only if they had been willing to let go of the 'sensation' of seeing inside would they have been able to start embracing or embodying the emotional, physical and mental aspects. Their clairvoyant abilities would have been even finer, more sensitive and definitely much healthier for them and those around them on many levels if they had been able to let go.

It was the same with my experience in India (described in Chapter 1). Only by letting go of the desire to see like this again was I able to get inside my visual pathway and gradually make my way to the other side. Sometimes it is necessary to let go of a treasured experience to find something better. For me it was essential to let go of the feeling of the experience from the past in India so that I could learn step-by-step how to get there and far beyond. The ability to direct myself is ultimately more important than the actual experience so that I am not dependent upon external circumstances for my internal state. Experiences are always different but the means of applying conscious depth perception is constant. In other words, learning and applying the principles is more important than the ever-changing experiences.

Meditation and the visual pathway

Many people comment that they are physically uncomfortable while meditating. I remember my own meditations in the past, associated with much pain and discomfort when sitting still. When I discovered and developed a means to stay within my visual pathway and direct myself in the meditation session from the upper visual cortex throughout the entire visual system, the pain and discomfort vanished, with no more mind wandering. And after an hour or so my eyes, vision, posture and mental attention are clear and focused. Meditation can become easy, enjoyable and pain-free.

I support people in their individual spiritual disciplines by helping them to apply conscious depth perception. This enables them to easily take care of their body and vision and to have inner time to direct their spiritual practices in daily life. Applying the principles will help the inside core of the brainstem and spinal cord to be more balanced while sitting, so that the person's sense of ease, peace and balance is easily maintained (see figures 7.23, 7.24 & 7.25).

On death and dying

In Japan one of my students asked me this question: "I have been practising Zen for over 10 years. When my spiritual practice goes well I feel that I am connected from somewhere behind and above the back of the skull. Then I feel I am rightly connected and grounded in my body. But when I concentrate on the space between my eyebrows I feel heavy, with pain in my body. Do you have any comments about this?"

If I connect with the space between my eyebrows I may try to 'get' something, but pain will be automatically mine, too. I will be using the frontal lobes for my thinking and 'thinking hard' will result in fatigue. This 'thinking hard' causes me to lose my overall coordination, which happens at the back of the skull.

On the other hand, the region behind and above the back of the skull is closely connected to the upper visual cortex, the place from which I would direct my conscious depth perception. It is the place some might call the 'doorway,' where we connect with a non-physical realm of guidance. This may well be the place from which we depart when we die. When I direct through my visual pathway from this place I am instantly connected with my physicality, and the body can be free.

If we have been primarily using our frontal lobes and our reptilian and limbic brains are

7.23 MEDITATION
with conscious depth perception

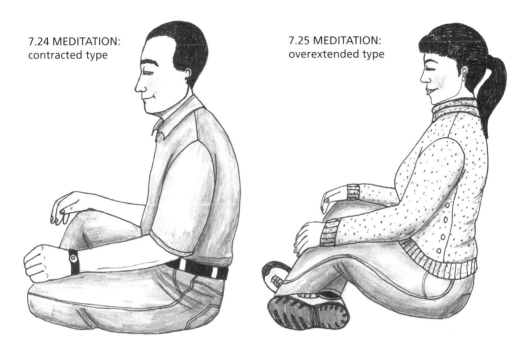

7.24 MEDITATION:
contracted type

7.25 MEDITATION:
overextended type

contracted, when we pass away we may take our unresolved emotions and visual images with us; we die in the same state in which we have lived. If we have lived life connected with the higher region of the visual pathway we can move through it and out this doorway through the upper visual cortex; leaving the body and staying conscious in the process of leaving. I would like to continue freeing my entire visual pathway so that in the process of passing away I may leave into total freedom without taking any unresolved emotional baggage with me. My intention is to work with this process now while I am living rather than waiting until I die.

Is this a luxury or a necessity?

It might seem like a luxury to learn to look after myself and to attend to my own vision to such an extent. On the other hand, this work is basic and necessary to prevent injury on perhaps many levels. For example, on a practical level many car accidents might be preventable if more people knew how to apply panoramic vision while driving. With panoramic vision the retina with its rods will be stimulated so that the body can respond simultaneously, more quickly, accurately and efficiently. Looking after myself is also ultimately beneficial to those around me, both directly and indirectly. Including my inner vision in my awareness will benefit my partner and children as well as my community as this will help me understand how best to communicate and participate in my relationships — and care for others when they need it. In addition, attending to my own overall health is of obvious benefit to those around me, as will be apparent to anyone who has ever tended a sick loved one. Learning to undo old emotional memories so that my inner state and my interactions with the people around me can flourish and thrive benefits us all.

The grandma who broke her glasses

In London I recently heard of an 81 year-old woman who broke her reading glasses. She had been wearing glasses since her 40s, but when she was in her early 80s her granddaughter, who told me the story, accidentally broke them. The grandmother did not replace her glasses but instead did all her sewing, reading and knitting for the 12 years until her death at age 93 without any visual aids.

Here's another heartening story from Switzerland; a woman had worn reading glasses for over 50 years. On her hundredth birthday she was so excited about all her greeting cards that she forgot to put on her glasses — she read all the cards without them. From that day on she didn't touch her glasses and could read and did all her other close activities with no vision aids.

*

It's never too late to change. At any age change can be accomplished. We have looked at the relationships between the body and eyes in different aspects of our lives where we can incorporate the visual system for better outcomes. The Eyebody Method can be easily integrated into our day-to-day activities: this is where it is needed. The following chapter explains how you can start the process of change.

8

First steps

There are many things you can do to begin to change your habits and bring awareness to your visual system. These include gradual steps to reduce the habit of wearing glasses or contact lenses, using pinhole glasses, activating the panoramic photoreceptors, and visual activities you can do on your own.

Take off your glasses and strengthen your visual system

Leaving your glasses off from time to time will help you become aware of when you really need them. Start noticing when it might not be necessary to use them. For instance if you wear glasses for myopia you don't need them for close-up reading; experiment with leaving them off. With presbyopia or hypermetropia you can see distant objects without glasses; perhaps leave them off when taking a walk. Start finding out when you don't really need them and when you do, even if the world is a little blurry. Don't be thrown by the belief that everything at all times has to be seen clearly. Wear glasses when you need them, like reading in dim light or driving a car. Just taking off your glasses from time to time will help undo habitual patterns, although the habit of effortful seeing or squinting to see may remain.

Often during workshops or individual lessons people ask me how to handle the process of changing the habit of wearing glasses. I usually design a programme for people which combines letting go of their glasses or contact lenses with learning how to use their overall visual system.

In a situation where no hands-on guidance is available I would start by asking: when is it really necessary for me to wear glasses?

In my teaching I guide people to find new solutions and make different choices. Often I notice that the feeling and belief of 'I can't do it' is stronger than the 'I can redirect the visual system so that seeing is effortless and clear.' The 'I can't do it' was not part of my own belief system, although for people who revert back to wearing glasses this may be a hindering thought pattern. In my teaching I work directly with this counterproductive thought form as its importance cannot be underestimated.

Transition glasses

Reducing the strength of prescription glasses for myopia, presbyopia and hypermetropia is a good step towards breaking the habit of wearing them. It gives the fovea centralis more room to function efficiently and naturally. By using appropriately reduced-strength glasses you are still legally able to drive (in the case of myopia). You may not see every tiny bird in the distance clearly, but this is not necessary while driving. The focusing of the light by the glasses, which overrides all subtle movement within the eye, will be directed a bit more towards the periphery of the fovea centralis rather than intensely focused on the centre. This will also give the brain more freedom and leeway to function. Remember from my own story that I had transition glasses 25% less than full-strength and I was able to see clearly through them after only one week. (This will differ from person to person and from situation to situation, so don't be disappointed if the change happens more slowly — or shocked if it happens more quickly).

Pinhole glasses — see more clearly while exercising the visual system from within

Pinhole glasses have pin-sized holes stamped out in black plastic (see figure 8.1). The specific size of the holes helps light reach the fovea centralis, where the cone photoreceptors send messages to the lower visual cortex for clear-sightedness. The result is similar to that of wearing normal prescription glasses. As an additional benefit, the blackness of the plastic helps stimulate the 95% of photoreceptors within the peripheral area of the retina (the rods — as in night vision) which send messages to the thalamus and to the upper visual cortex. This means the all-essential panoramic vision is stimulated.

You can wear them during many activities, including reading, writing, computing, watching television or a movie, or going for a walk. This will help you to see more clearly and to exercise the visual system intrinsically. Wearing them for periods in the garden or on the beach (but not while driving, as your responses may not be as fast as you need) will also help.

Depending on how visually fatigued you are, the holes may appear very small if you are of the contracted upper visual cortex type. When your retina increases its efficiency, with more panoramic photoreceptors responding, the holes will seem bigger. It can seem as if there is only one hole per eye — and everything looks very clear and well defined.

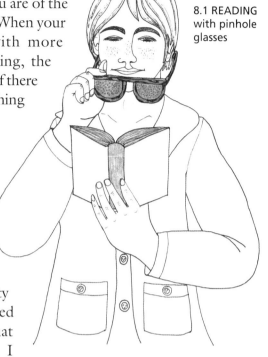

8.1 READING with pinhole glasses

When I first started to wear pinholes I was unable to see through the holes and got dizzy. But I persevered and after some weeks, as my retina changed, the rods became more stimulated and lively and my experience changed completely, to the point where I could see with the same clarity as with any glasses. The holes looked bigger and bigger — an indicator that the retina was fully functioning. I continue using pinhole glasses as an intrinsic exercise tool from time to time, even though I now see clearly.

When you begin wearing pinhole glasses don't overuse them. Start with 5-10 minutes. As with anything else, it's good to start slowly and increase the time gradually. Should it feel emotionally uncomfortable to use them, take heart: as the retina improves so does the comfort.

Not all pinhole glasses are the same. There are different makes and brands — some better than others. If the holes are too small not enough light will reach the retina; if the holes are too large too much light falls onto the outer edge of the macula. I recommend glasses with round holes rather than square, as the retina is round. Use only plastic and not glass, as glass bends the light and produces a different effect on the retina. (For pinhole glasses you can trust see the back of this book.)

While you are wearing your pinhole glasses, remember to develop awareness from the panoramic area of the retina (for contracted types) or from the lower visual cortex (for overextended types). This is what will make the fundamental difference — something you take with you once you take the pinhole glasses off.

The stages of learning this method

There are three stages of learning this process. The first is the distinction between focused and panoramic vision; the second is embodying the visual pathways with conscious depth perception and changing habitual ways of seeing; the third is applying conscious depth perception to the visual pathways and extending that to the environment in everyday life. For the second stage and the beginning of the third stage, we need a teacher. For the first stage I am including some activities you can do on your own.

The first step is to discover the difference between panoramic and focused vision. This you can experience for yourself on your own. You can apply panoramic vision: to the activities of palming and sunning (directions follow on pages 114-16) as well as to reading this book or any activity in your life. Proceeding in this way does not incorporate the overall coordinating mechanism, but these are useful and necessary beginning steps.

It's a matter of taking it step-by-step; that is the easiest way to get to the mountain top — and safely back again.

I recommend you record your experiences. This is a good way to increase your awareness and track your progress.

The first step — panoramic vision

Overextended and contracted upper visual cortex types each require different specific directions, but in the end we come to the same integration of the visual system. Follow the directions for the character type relevant to you. If you are overextended on one side of your visual cortex and contracted on the other side (myopic in one eye and hypermetropic in the other), follow the steps for the contracted type first, then proceed with the overextended instructions.

By focused vision I mean primarily using the fovea centralis (the centre of the retina) which has about 5% of all photoreceptors; by panoramic vision I mean using the over 95% of the retina surrounding the fovea centralis which includes the rest of the photoreceptors. The panoramic area of the retina is not stimulated when we 'just 100% focus' on an object. Nor do we stimulate the panoramic area when we wear prescription glasses.

The purpose of the following activity is to distinguish between focused and panoramic vision. Over the long-term we would like to include both in an appropriate fashion in our daily activities.

For the contracted type:

1. Please take off your glasses or take out your contact lenses. Welcome to the blur! Remember that when I first consciously took off my glasses in the beginning I could not see more than about 10 cm in front of my eyes. Give yourself time.

2. Now, without your glasses, either walk around or if seated just look around. Do this somewhere safe and familiar. You may feel embarrassed, strange, anxious — notice this. If appropriate, let people know you are working on your eyes and vision.

3. Be attentive to the inside of your eyes and mentally step back into the inside depth of the retina and the surrounding layer of the choroid. The retina is the inner layer of your eye and spans from the back of your eye all the way to the pupil spherically towards the front of your eye. The retina has multiple layers of photoreceptors and the choroid process is just behind. Get a sense of the panoramic vision from inside your retina. From the back of your brain, visualise expanding your retina and choroid three-dimensionally all the way to the pupil in the front of your eye. Practise this for 30 seconds to a minute; allow your thoughts to widen the retina and choroid. Notice while you practise how you feel emotionally, physically and mentally.

4. Now focus on an object and walk towards it, using focused vision only. Notice how it feels emotionally, physically, mentally.

5. Do this again, this time begin by using your panoramic vision for 30 seconds.

6. Notice the differences and if you wish, write them down. What was it like? Did you notice anything about your body? Did you notice anything about your eyes? How did you feel emotionally? What was your mental attitude?

7. Practise panoramic vision as you walk or look around, then after 30 seconds include attentiveness from your lower visual cortex to make contact with the objects. Notice what this feels like.

I suggest you practise panoramic vision from within your retina and choroids frequently in your daily activities — while reading this book, brushing your teeth or eating your dinner. Bring it into your daily life and as well notice when you don't. Become aware of the difference.

For the overextended type:

1. Be attentive to your lower visual cortex. Gradually allow panoramic vision to emerge from within the lower visual cortex. You may notice a release of unnecessary tension by letting go of over-focusing. Give yourself time. Notice how you feel physically, emotionally, mentally.

2. Now focus on an object and walk towards it, using focused vision only. Notice how it feels emotionally, physically, mentally.

3. Walk towards an object again, this time using panoramic vision from the lower visual cortex.

4. Notice the differences and if you wish, write them down. What was it like? Did you notice anything about your body? Did you notice anything about your eyes? How did you feel emotionally? What was your mental attitude?

5. Practise using panoramic vision from the lower visual cortex — that is, letting go of over-focusing — in your daily activities. Notice especially what happens when objects, people or events come closer.

Palming

Palming helps stimulate panoramic vision and release eyestrain (see figure 8.2).

Palming for contracted types:

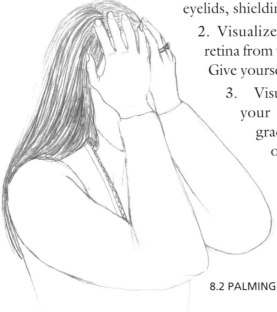

1. Place the palms of your hands over your closed eyelids, shielding off the light.

2. Visualize panoramic space within your retina from the back of the retina to the pupil. Give yourself time to think, to visualize this.

3. Visualize your choroid layer behind your retina filled with blood which gradually moves forwards past the ora serrata to the pupils. Again, give yourself time.

4. Notice your vitreous humour, the jelly-like fluid within your eyeball. Allow this vitreous humour fluid to be alive. Notice you can move this

8.2 PALMING

fluid by visualizing it. Make contact with your eyeball towards the back of your eye (which is elongated if you are myopic) with this fluid. Let it back off your lens; give it more room to support the retina all around.

5. Alternate this activity with that of Sunning (see below) in intervals of around two to three minutes.

Palming for overextended types:

1. Place the palms of your hands over your closed eyelids, shielding off the light.

2. Be attentive to your lower visual cortex. Gradually allow panoramic vision to emerge from within the lower visual cortex. You may notice a release of unnecessary tension by letting go of over-focusing. Give yourself time. Renew this intention frequently while you palm.

3. Alternate this activity with that of Sunning (see below) in intervals of about two to three minutes.

'Sunning' stimulates the entire retina, thalamus and hypothalamus

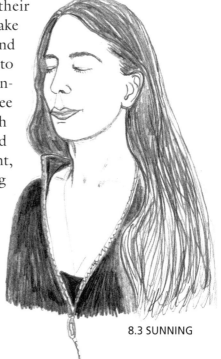

One purpose of sunning is to stimulate the thalamus and hypothalamus and their respective glands. In sunning you take your hands off your closed eyelids and move your head delicately from side to side, ideally facing the sun, or altern-atively a source of light like a lamp (see figure 8.3). Continue throughout with closed eyelids. Turn your head (and therefore your eyes) towards the light, only as much as you can without feeling like you have to resist or tighten against it. If you are sensitive to light you may not be able to face too much light right away, but this will change in a short amount of time if you stick with it.

8.3 SUNNING

For contracted types:

1. Through your closed eyelids visualize the sun's rays stimulating the panoramic photoreceptors within your retina and allow the choroid behind the retina to fill with fluid from the back all the way to the pupil in the front.

2. Alternate this with Palming two or three times, doing each for two or three minutes at a time.

Notice after each practice how you feel emotionally, how you see close-up and in the distance, how you experience colour. Notice your body.

For overextended types:

1. With your eyelids closed, visualize panoramic vision from within the lower visual cortex as you face the sun. Give yourself time. Notice the light entering even through closed eyelids.

2. Alternate this with Palming two or three times, doing each for two or three minutes at a time.

Refining the kinaesthetic sense of the visual system

While we are all made up of bones, tissue and muscles and affected by Eyebody Patterns and upper visual cortex type regardless of culture, socio-economic status and childhood upbringing, we are all unique.

An individualized approach is vital as we all think, see and feel somewhat differently. Guided principle-based processes are essential to connect us with our own overall mechanisms, so that we can apply the learning to our own specific visual system and situation.

We must remember that habits develop over many years and often we don't recognize them as habits. They become the norm. Anything different we may consider very strange. Here the guided process becomes essential.

Conclusions

The steps to letting go of glasses or contact lenses completely and waking up the whole visual system are coupled with a developing sense of the visual pathways and the process of seeing in daily activities. The body and the eye will automatically follow with an increase of visual system function and coordination. Deciding how and when to use glasses is a first step, followed by wearing transition glasses if necessary. Pinhole glasses can be used to stimulate the retina and the pathways to the thalamus, while allowing you to see objects more clearly.

Alternating between 'Palming' and 'Sunning' vision activities helps harmonize photoreceptor function, opens the pathways to the thalamus and strengthens the intrinsic awareness of the eyes and lower visual cortex. This is a beginning…

9

Future possibilities

When we wear glasses or contact lenses we alter our natural state of being and limit possibilities. We also subtly influence the way our brain works. Not only that, but as we have seen with the Eyebody Patterns we are also influencing our physicality and the functioning of our organs and nervous system, along with our emotional behaviour and mental processes. These are far-reaching effects. Yet most of the time we put on glasses without thinking of effects they may have on how we are feeling and functioning right now.

By tapping into our innate intelligence, our inner knowing, we can learn to coordinate our visual pathways, whether of the contracted or overextended type.

My experiences in India allowed me to see myself and the world around me very differently. Suddenly losing this heightened awareness of seeing motivated me to start asking questions about vision, to discover and then learn to apply new techniques to my seeing in daily life. This freed me from the habit of wearing glasses and step-by-step improved the functioning of my entire visual system. This has given me a deep sense of safety in knowing that the ability to fully see and function is mine for life. You too can experience this.

I have minutely observed my own processes and progress with this work. I could have missed that first small experience of the cornea relating to the chest area of my body. But being in the right mental space at the right time, I became aware of the importance of this seemingly innocuous occurrence. It has changed my mental outlook and inside awareness forever. Becoming more and more interested in the relationship between the eyes and the body and experimenting widely has allowed me to see the relationships very clearly.

Over years of experimenting I have noticed more and more subtle relationships occurring within the brain, eyes and body. I have gradually discovered the access routes into my own brain, stimulating it and improving my overall functioning. The realization that the function of the thalamus is also directly linked to the visual system has led to the understanding that our entire emotional, physical, mental and spiritual well-being depends on an optimally-functioning visual system. The key to achieving this is conscious depth perception within the upper visual cortex.

At times I wondered if this was all only in my own head. Could others learn this? Was I able to communicate this process clearly and find out where other people were in their own awareness? The answer has been yes. When I started to work with other people I realized my findings were generalisable and that it was possible for people to work with their own visual systems as I did with mine. For people of all ages this work can help them let go of glasses, prevent the build-up of tensions within the visual pathway and the body, and help develop new pathways for better functioning and coordination. As I keep on learning and teaching I realize the scope of this work is far wider than I ever anticipated.

If we educate children to be in touch with their panoramic vision from an early age, it may help them grow up more coordinated, less fatigued and more socially aware. The ability to learn from within, to visualize, will help them develop to their highest potential. This process will enhance their individual well-being as well as the well-being of those around them.

As human beings we are not islands and there is an increasing need to extend our vision beyond ourselves personally to encompass our home, work, school and community environments, our national and international surroundings and the people living in them.

There are two environments I have to take care of: my inner environment, and my immediate surrounding environment. By using conscious depth perception from the upper visual cortex, I will be better able to take care of both. Let's say I have to deal with a group of five people, or an audience of five thousand. First I bring my attention inside. I come back to my upper visual cortex for overall coordination, direction and inspiration so that I can take care of my brainstem and spinal cord without interfering in their processes. I tune into my visual system so that all the parts of my eyes — and my brain and body — can function effectively and efficiently. Only then do I take in the outer environment of the room and the audience, using panoramic vision which allows me to both have an overview of the entire environment as well as attend to details. That is all I have to do; see and take care. The situations will be different — it might be my rowdy teenage children, or my dying grandmother, or the business meeting where important decisions have to be made. Situations change from moment to moment, but the same principles and processes apply. What I have to do is learn to attend to myself first, then include my environment with panoramic vision and attentiveness to detail.

From whatever entry point you come to this work — a desire to let go of glasses or contact lenses and to see clearly naturally, to improve your personal health, release tension in your eyes and body, improve overall coordination, or specific body use — this work of coordinating and integrating your visual system and using it effectively and efficiently will help you achieve your goals. You are likely to experience other possibilities not previously imagined towards enriching the quality of your life.

For me this is only the beginning of a new way of working on the human development frontier with far-reaching possibilities and outcomes for the individual and wider community. This whole organic unfolding of a process of discovery and methods of learning and teaching is by no means completed. Deeper understandings of the intrinsic Eyebody Patterns will unfold.

In the realm of applying the principles in life's activities, the scope and applications are never-ending and infinite. The quality of my life has improved with increased clarity, health and awareness in my inner and outer environment without the use of glasses, contact lenses or laser surgery. I would like to extend to you the possibility of benefiting in the same way.

You do not have to change the things you are doing in your life; just change and thus enhance the way you are doing them. Don't give up any disciplines that are helping you: meditation, psychotherapy, cranial osteopathy, yoga, Alexander Technique, whatever they may be. Keep on with the activities you enjoy, like reading, singing, running, or cycling.

Learn to apply the principles described in this book, and notice the difference. You will find that when your visual system is functioning properly there is an increased sense of ease — and increased enjoyment in all your activities. You will also find that there is better overall efficiency and effectiveness in whatever you are doing.

The intelligence of our visual system is accessible regardless of the activity in which we are engaged — even while our eyelids are closed while we are asleep. We can ignore it, but this will not help us gain inner freedom. If we consistently apply the principles outlined in this book to all our activities, the result will be better coordination, increased efficiency, increased mental attentiveness, clearer communication, a change for the better for our environment and those around us — and finally, the enjoyment of being truly in the present moment.

Frequently asked questions

Here are answers to some common questions about the Eyebody Method. An in-depth answer to each question can be found in the body of the book.

Can this work help me?

This method can help anyone who is interested in investigating and improving their eyesight, vision, body, emotional balance and brain function.

What is this Method about?

I have discovered direct links between parts of the eyes, the brain and the body. I call these links the Eyebody Patterns. The visual system has multiple functions aside from our eyesight and therefore is a reliable tool for the guidance and oversight of our entire self.

The methods help us consciously direct the visual system, stimulating new pathways in the brain and releasing tensions held in the visual system and the body simultaneously. They can reduce and eliminate the need for glasses or contact lenses and maintain good vision.

What is the visual system?

The visual system includes all areas in the eyes and brain which are associated in the widest sense with receiving light, transforming the incoming information and making sense of it.

The upper visual pathway passes through the reptilian brain (fight and flight), the limbic system (emotions), and the neocortex (conscious and factual thinking). Coordinating these parts of the brain is fundamental to making any lasting changes in the visual system.

What comes first — eye or body dysfunctions?

Like the chicken and egg question, the two are interrelated. My experience is that visual dysfunctions are established first, sometimes subtly and without our knowledge. Because this deterioration can be quite gradual, the experience of either visual blurring or physical discomfort often presents itself years after the initial dysfunction begins. The pattern always seems to be found in both the visual system and the body as a whole — the systems mirror one another.

What are the differences between principles and exercises?

Principles are concepts, which apply regardless of the activity or situation. Exercises are activities associated with some form of 'doing' or physical action. The Method uses visual principles which allow the brain, eye and body to function more easily as a coordinated whole. These principles can then be applied to any activity, such as reading the newspaper, driving a car, walking, and 'eye exercises' themselves.

Does this Method help every condition?

Generally speaking, yes. It is possible to change most eye or body problems by gradually working with and coordinating the entire visual system. Specific visual and physical conditions will, over time, improve and begin to function naturally and optimally.

Will it help in cases of short-sightedness, middle-age vision, far-sightedness from an early age and astigmatism?

Yes. These are common visual malfunctions. By learning to release tension within the visual system the physiology of each condition changes.

The areas of the body likely to be affected by these conditions are:

1. **Short-sightedness (myopia)** affects the lower back and pelvic area, the upper legs to the knees. It can also cause neck and shoulder tension, with a general postural slump.

2. **Middle-age vision (presbyopia)** also affects the lower back and pelvis as well as the upper back, chest area and the breathing mechanism.

3. **Far-sightedness (hypermetropia)** affects the upper area of the body, especially the heart and lung region. This can be emotionally manifested as short temper, and impatience with oneself and others.

4. **Astigmatism** affects the shoulder girdle and neck region with a slumping of the shoulders

Will the Method help glaucoma, cataracts or macular degeneration?

Yes, in all three conditions the overall activity of the visual brain needs to be increased first through conscious depth perception. Eye improvements will follow.

10.1 CROSS-EYES WITH BODY CONNECTING

Notice how the legs rotate in the same direction as the eye

Eye See — Vision Issue; Direction — A Journal on the Alexander Technique. Vol 2 No 7. Sydney: Fyncot Pty Ltd, 1999

Will it help with crossed-eyes?

Yes, in most cases. Crossed-eyes have to do with disruptions in the connections of the optic nerves to the brainstem and the overall upper visual cortex functions. This can be rectified so that both visual pathways function together.

Crossed-eyes manifest physically in the lower limbs; the affected side of the upper leg will turn either in or out, impacting the legs, the knees, and their connection to the pelvis.

Can physical problems and postural misalignment be corrected and discomfort reduced?

In most cases, yes. The eyes and their connections to the brain provide us with a map of our physical problems. The Method will address these problems: first indirectly by applying general principles, and then directly through improving the functioning of the visual system. The rest of the body responds simultaneously.

If you struggle with physical, mental or emotional difficulty or pain, it is possible that these malfunctions have yet to manifest themselves visually. Resolving these issues can help ensure clear sight for years to come.

Is it possible for me to stop wearing my glasses?

Yes, in most cases this is absolutely possible. Depending on your commitment and how conscientiously you apply the Method, you can let go of your glasses or contact lenses. This process varies in length; for some it is shorter, for some longer, depending on such factors as the weakness of the visual system, and attachment to the habit of wearing glasses.

What is involved in letting go of glasses?

It involves two processes: letting go of the habit of wearing glasses and simultaneously strengthening the visual system.

For some people I might suggest using reduced-strength lenses so that the transition is easier. By applying the Method your visual system will gradually improve, and the need for glasses or contacts will diminish.

How long before I can go without glasses/contacts altogether?

This depends on the nature of your eyesight difficulty, your readiness to change your habits, and your ability to apply the principles. In activities like driving and reading, the process can be fun and enjoyable if you take it step-by-step.

If I have already had an operation, can the Method help me?

Yes. If an operation was performed, let's say for crossed-eyes in childhood, cataracts, or retinal detachment, you can learn to use your visual system better and prevent either further deterioration or a recurrence. Generally an operation compromises the whole visual system by permanently changing the structure of part of the eye. Learning to use the visual system in a more efficient way helps ensure that no further surgery will be needed and that any physical changes occurring to compensate will not create an additional problem.

If I have had refractive laser surgery to improve my eyesight can I benefit from the Method?

Laser surgery is performed on the cornea so that the light will fall directly onto the fovea centralis, resulting in clear-sight. However, the 'condition' of the visual dysfunction (the elongated or shortened eyeball) and the habitual use of the visual brain still remain.

Although you might not wear glasses any longer and be satisfied, you can learn how to use the whole visual system fully and more efficiently.

Sometimes the operation is not completely successful. If you still need glasses (perhaps 20/20 was not achieved), or develop another malfunction (such as lack of clarity reading close-up or increased light sensitivity), the Method will help you learn how to handle your condition naturally and safely from within.

Will my vision and body posture improve at the same rate?

Yes, although posture may appear to improve more rapidly because we are more accustomed to observing the body than the subtleties of our vision.

What is required for me to start learning this Method?

There are few basic requirements. A certain level of commitment and willingness to change is fundamental. It's important to keep an open mind when learning something new. A constructive scepticism can be helpful but a destructive scepticism will not allow you to learn; it will limit you to what you already know.

Is there an age at which I should start learning? Is age a factor?

The learning process is not dependent on age. You are never too young or too old.

Can this method still help someone in their 70s or 80s?

Certainly. I have had people in my retreats in their 90s who did very well. Age is not a limitation, and change may or may not be slower. I notice that age can sometimes be a big advantage, as life experience helps to make one more observant, and often more thoughtful and aware.

How long will it take me to learn this?

That depends on different factors: the ability to learn kinaesthetically as well as conceptually; a certain openness and readiness; commitment to changing your attentiveness in daily activities; and the ability to apply the principles to daily activities will all play a part in how quickly you learn.

Can pre-birth conditions be reversed?

Yes they can. We continue to grow and change even after we leave the womb. Conditions in place when we were born can be gradually changed.

What is the relationship between emotions and vision?

Emotions like anxiety, fear or anger play a large role in our vision. The vitreous humour fluid (the fluid within the eyeball) plays a major role in the balance of emotions (and is also associated with the lower back region), as well as the limbic system (the emotional brain) which stores old pictures and experiences. By releasing the vitreous humor, the jelly like fluid within the eyeball, emotions are eased and the lower back and visceral organs will gradually function more normally. Coordinating the limbic system will also help to release 'old pictures' without having to name any of the associated experiences.

Are there any benefits apart from improved eyesight and posture?

Participants frequently comment on other benefits. They report gaining a feeling of lightness, less anxiety (especially in short-sightedness), less pain in menstrual cycles and increased attention and mental clarity.

The overall increase in brain activity stimulates brain, eye and body functioning and therefore the overall health of a person improves.

What are the benefits of individual lessons?

Individual lessons can be useful and are offered in certain locations when available. The combination of individual lessons and workshop attendance is the best way to assimilate, learn and practise with support from others.

Self-help is always encouraged. However, when we work with life-long habits it is easier to be guided by a skilled teacher who has been there before. Together you can discover new ways to think and respond and thereby recognize old habits to freely choose what is appropriate — rather than be stuck in old habits.

How do pinhole glasses help?

Pinhole glasses are an excellent tool for seeing clearly and exercising the panoramic as well as the macular area of the retina within the eye. Start using them for watching TV, going to the movies, or reading. They help in cases of short-sightedness, far-sightedness, astigmatism, and middle-age sight.

When can I start applying the Method in my personal daily activities?

Right now, in activities such as reading the paper or working at the computer, driving a car or washing dishes. It will become fun to observe yourself and learn to function with more ease and clarity.

Can I apply the principles in my professional life and my recreational activities?

Absolutely yes. If you use a computer you will notice a change in the way you use your brain, eyes and body. In sports or workouts you will see an increase in your potential as you use the visual process to enhance what you have already achieved. If you are a musician you will gradually be able to apply this to your ability to read sheet music and perform.

Learning by participating in retreat workshops

The first step is often participating in a retreat workshop. These are run annually in different parts of the world. Group and individual attention is given to learn and practise the principles and to assimilate them gradually. Sharing in the experiences of others helps the learning process.

REFERENCES

Alexander, FM, *The Use of the Self*. London: Victor Gollancz Ltd, 1985

Alexander, FM, *Constructive Conscious Control of the Individual*. London: Victor Gollancz Ltd, 1987

Bates, WH, *Better Eyesight without Glasses*. New York: Henry Holt & Co, 1981

Bennis, Warren and Nanus, Bert, *Leaders: The Strategies for Taking Charge*. New York: Harper & Row, 1985

Garlick, David, *The Lost Sixth Sense, A Medical Scientist Looks at the Alexander Technique*. New South Wales: University of New South Wales, 1990

Goodrich, Janet, *Natural Vision Improvement*. Berkeley: Celestial Arts, 1986

Goodrich, Janet, *Help your child to perfect eyesight without glasses*. Burra Creek, New South Wales: Sally Milner Publishing Pty Ltd, 1996

Grunwald, Peter (issue editorial), *Eye See — Vision Issue; Direction — A Journal on the Alexander Technique. Vol 2 No 7*. Sydney: Fyncot Pty Ltd, 1999

Hubel, David, *Eye, Brain and Vision*. New York: Scientific American Library, 1995.

Huxley, Aldous, *The Art of Seeing*. New York: Harper & Brothers, 1942

Upledger, John E, *Craniosacral Therapy Two: Beyond the Dura*. Seattle: Eastland Press, Inc, 1987

GLOSSARY OF TERMS

H ere is an explanation of some Eyebody terms that have been used in this book.

Conscious depth perception is a visual direction, a conscious thinking/ visualizing process from the upper visual cortex that coordinates and integrates all aspects of the visual system and the brain.

Eyebody Patterns are a map of the human body within the visual system that show the connections between different areas of the brain, the eyes and the body.

Focused vision is using the fovea centralis (the centre of the retina within the macula) exclusively. It is associated with details, clarity, high-resolution sight and colour perception.

Panoramic vision is a visual direction, a conscious thinking/visualizing process to access consciously the upper visual pathway thereby stimulating new pathways in the brain.

Primary coordinating mechanism is one of the Eyebody Principles. Housed in the upper visual cortex and stimulated through conscious depth perception, it coordinates the multiple functions of the visual system and therefore the whole self.

Upper visual cortex character or type (the overextended or contracted) describes the predominant upper visual cortex tendency with which we are born. This determines our overall visual functioning, underlies any visual dysfunction, and is the source of many of our personality traits.

Visual cortex is divided into the lower visual cortex and upper visual cortex. The lower visual cortex, responsible for high definition, focused vision and colour perception, is traditionally called the striate cortex or primary visual cortex. The upper visual cortex is associated with conscious, three-dimensional thinking and houses the primary coordinating mechanism, which is activated through conscious depth perception.

Visual fatigue is a general weakness within the visual system.

Visual pathways (upper and lower) are the conduits for information from the eyes to the upper and lower visual cortex. The visual pathway specifically refers to the parts of the visual system between the eyes and the visual cortex.

Visual radiation is divided into lower and upper visual radiation and refers to areas of the visual system information passes through just before it reaches the visual cortex. The lower visual radiation is the region of fibres where the information passes from the lateral geniculate bodies to the lower visual cortex. The upper visual radiation is associated with the area of the limbic system from the third ventricle via the fornix, the limbic fluid and through the corpus callosum.

Visual system consists of all areas (intrinsic and extrinsic) of the eye, the lower and upper visual pathways and the lower and upper visual cortex. The visual system is present in each part of the brain: reptilian, limbic and neocortex and can be coordinated by means of conscious depth perception.

INDEX

A

Alexander, Frederick Mathias 14, 19, 45-6, 50

Alexander Technique 8-9, 11, 14, 19, 33, 45, 47-8, 102, 120

amygdala 26-7, 84

anti-social disconnection 84

anxiety 18, 21, 23, 42, 62-3, 84-5, 92-3, 96, 113, 126-7

aqueous humour 28, 30-1, 40, 65, 71-2, 74, 83-4, 86, 88-9

astigmatism 9, 12-13, 16, 20, 33, 39, 42, 48, 55, 57, 62-3, 69-71, 86, 123, 127

auto-immune difficulties 82

auxiliary eye 29

B

back pain 12, 55, 58, 79, 82, 87

Barstow, Marjory 19

Bates Method of Natural Vision 9, 12, 14

Bates, William H 14

blood circulation 30, 45, 71, 76, 86, 88

blurry eyesight 16, 22, 31, 33, 41, 58, 65, 68, 109

BodyMind Centering 9

Brain Gym 12

brainstem 25-6, 30, 42, 52, 56, 64, 92-3, 97, 99, 101, 106, 119, 124

breathing 36, 40, 44, 50, 55, 63, 65-7, 73-4, 80, 86, 93, 95, 97, 123

breathing problems 12, 55

Brenner, William 20

C

canal of Schlemm 40, 71-2, 88

cataracts 13, 20, 39-40, 42, 55, 72-4, 86, 123, 125

chiasm, *see* optic chiasm

children 40, 93, 119

chiropractic 48, 63, 70, 79

choroid 30, 35, 42, 57, 60-2, 71, 74, 76-9, 81, 86-8, 96, 100-1, 113-14, 116

ciliary body 30, 86, 88

ciliary process 30, 65

colour perception 29-30, 130

communication 19-20, 38, 48, 51, 56, 58, 91-3, 119, 121

computing 38, 54, 63-4, 80, 90, 94-6, 110, 127

conjunctiva 28-9, 34, 60, 79-80, 85-6, 89

conscious depth perception 11, 37, 44, 49-66 *passim*, 80, 83, 88, 90, 93-106 *passim*, 112, 119, 123, 130-1

contact lenses 9, 20, 22, 33, 37, 43, 57-8, 61, 63, 96-7, 99-100, 109, 113, 116, 118, 120, 122, 124-5

contracted character 39, 41-3, 51, 57, 65-6, 70, 73, 80, 85, 92-6, 98-101, 103, 107, 111-14, 116, 118, 130

cornea 8, 13, 27-31, 33-4, 40, 48, 59-60, 65, 69-71, 79-80, 86, 88, 118, 125

corpus callosum 26-7, 37, 60, 69-70, 86, 88, 131

cross-eyes 13, 39-40, 74-5, 87, 124-5

RESOURCES AND CONTACT INFORMATION

The eyebody.com website brings you up to date with retreat schedules and bookings, retreat venues, consultations, resources and more information.

As outlined in this book I recommend the use of pinhole glasses.

Three styles are available:

MEN'S
(dark brown, larger frame)

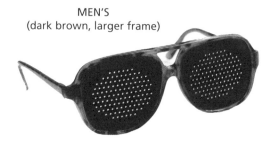

WOMEN'S
(dark brown)

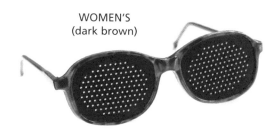

UNISEX
(light gray, smaller frame)

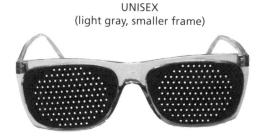

Books and pinhole glasses can be ordered directly through the website, by email, post, phone or fax. Retail or other inquiries should also be directed to:

Grunwald & Associates
The Eyebody Method®
PO Box 46 325
Herne Bay
Auckland
New Zealand
Phone +64 9 360 1730
Fax +64 9 360 1720
Email info@eyebody.com
Website www.eyebody.com

*